Board Work

Dennis D. Pointer
James E. Orlikoff

Foreword by
Stephen M. Shortell, Ph.D.

Board Work

Governing Health Care Organizations

Jossey-Bass Publishers
San Francisco
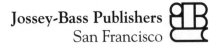

Jossey-Bass books and products are available through most bookstores. To contact Jossey-Bass directly, call (888) 378-2537, fax to (800) 605-2665, or visit our
website at www.josseybass.com.

Substantial discounts on bulk quantities of Jossey-Bass books are available to
corporations, professional associations, and other organizations. For details and
discount information, contact the special sales department at Jossey-Bass.

Library of Congress Cataloging-in-Publication Data

Pointer, Dennis Dale.
      Board work: governing health care organizations/Dennis D. Pointer, James E.
  Orlikoff; foreword by Stephen M. Shortell.—1st ed.
         p. cm.
  Includes bibliographical references and index.
  ISBN 0-7879-4299-5 (alk. paper)
  1. Health facilities—Administration. 2. Hospital trustees. 3. Boards of directors.
  I. Orlikoff, James E. II. Title.
  RA971.P626 1999
  362.1'068'4—dc21   99-19930

FIRST EDITION
HB Printing   10 9 8 7 6 5 4

Contents

List of Exhibits

Foreword

The health care sector has become increasingly complex, reflecting a turbulence of actions and reactions seldom seen before. The growth of public and private sector managed care has resulted in increased concerns about quality and outcomes of care and new demands for evidence-based accountability. Greater financial risk is being transferred directly to providers. The lines of division between hospitals, health systems, physician groups, and insurance plans are becoming more permeable, reflecting both vertical and virtual relationships. While providers continue to pursue various ways of reinventing themselves, over forty million Americans remain uninsured.

The U.S. health care system is in a critical stage of transformation. At its heart is a redefinition of—and search for—value. Value can be created in two ways: an organization can provide a service of a given quality level at a lower cost than its competitors, or it can provide a service of greater quality for a given cost—quality in both cases being defined in terms of criteria desired by the prospective purchaser. In the U.S. health care system, value has been created in the past primarily through investment in physical assets. In the future, value is more likely to be created through investment in information assets, knowledge-building assets, and relationship-building assets. A premium will be placed on intellectual capital fueled by information systems and the Internet and much greater attention will be given to the customer and to communities served.

Most health care organizations do not understand how they currently create value or how they will create value in the future. While executives and health care professionals must assume their fair share of responsibility for this, authors Dennis Pointer and James Orlikoff rightly highlight the failure of governance of our health care organizations. Many if not most governing board members do not really understand either the organization they purport to govern or the health care environment in which that organization exists.

Incremental improvement in board structure, composition, skills, or processes will not do the job. What is needed is a total rethinking of the governance concept and the implications that this holds for governance work—just the approach you'll find in this book.

Board Work is the best book on health care organization governance that I have ever read. These authors pull no punches. They provide a candid assessment of the current failures of health care governance. But this is not a negative book. The authors present a detailed, constructive approach for radically changing the current state of affairs.

The book lays out a visionary and detailed road map for governance transformation. Beginning with a fundamental consideration of stakeholders, it goes on to suggest a series of principles, practices, assessment tools, and recommendations to achieve breakthroughs in governance performance. Particularly valuable is the development of a governance assessment instrument, the results of which can be turned into a map that identifies performance gaps. For each gap, the authors suggest a practical program of action for improvement.

While it is clear that the health system faces many challenges that will not be solved by improved governance alone, it is also clear that these challenges will not be successfully addressed without radically improved governance. The authors have laid out both the challenge and an action plan. The hope is that current and future

trustees will have the courage to step up to the plate and begin to
lead their organizations toward the creation of greater value, rather
than settling for the largely reactionary behavior that marks many
current efforts.

March 1999   STEPHEN M. SHORTELL, PH.D.
                         Blue Cross of California Distinguished Professor
                         of Health Policy and Management,
                         Division of Health Policy and Management,
                         School of Public Health
                         Professor of Organization Behavior,
                         Haas School of Business,
                         University of California, Berkeley

Preface

Board work is tough and important work; it is done by part-time volunteers who must direct and oversee large and incredibly complex organizations operating in an industry and markets undergoing profound change. The work of boards has significant consequences for the viability of institutions providing critical services having a massive impact on community health and well-being.

Over the last twenty years we have worked with hundreds of health care organization boards and thousands of board members. Boards that want to really govern; dedicated, talented board members who devote incredible amounts of time and effort doing so. Yet the performance and contributions of most boards can be dramatically improved. Here are some of the biggest barriers we have encountered:

- A board's foundational obligation is to represent the interests of stakeholders (stockholders in for-profit entities). Yet many boards have not explicitly identified key stakeholders and do not have a good sense of what these groups want from, and expect of, their organizations.
- Many boards, and board members, do not have an empowering notion of the type of work they should be doing to make the greatest difference. As a consequence boards often focus too much attention, time, and effort on peripheral matters where they add

little value, rather than on issues where they can and must make significant contributions.

•   Governance structures—particularly in nonprofit health care systems—are often overweight, cumbersome, and fragmented. Most have too many boards, board committees, and meetings. Proposals and recommendations must wind their way through a governance labyrinth that significantly decreases an organization's strategic and operational metabolic rate at a time when decisiveness and agility are needed most.

•   Board meeting time is often spent mainly on passively listening to reports and receiving background information—from management, the medical staff, and the board's own committees. Little time is left for the "red meat" of governing: deliberating and debating decisions and policies that require board input and action.

•   Boards are rarely provided the type of information they need to govern—and they rarely have a clear enough picture of what they need to demand it.

Pause and Reflect: Your Board

If you are feeling this is a tad bit harsh, think about your own board:

• Has your board explicitly identified the organization's key stakeholders? Who are they? To what extent do you and your colleagues fully understand these stakeholders' interests and what they want and expect?

• What degree of consensus is there among members regarding the type of work your board should be doing? Does your board have a job description that specifically lays out its responsibilities, roles, and duties?

• How much of your board's attention is focused on matters that are peripheral to the organization's ability to fulfill its vision and mission?

• Does your board discuss and make conscious choices regarding the most significant and important issues it must address—and then structure its meeting agendas accordingly?

- What percentage of board meeting time do you spend sitting and listening (to reports and the presentation of background information) versus deliberating and debating important issues?

- Have you stopped reading large portions your board's meeting agenda packets because the materials are out of focus, poorly summarized, or just plain irrelevant?

We are tough on boards because we recognize their importance and know how great they can be.

Boards are as high up in an organization as one can go and still remain inside it (Carver, 1991). They are where the buck stops. Boards, what they do and how they do it, make an enormous difference. This book is for those who are serious about governing. Our audience is governance's front line: board members, board chairs, and CEOs. This book will provide you with a host of practical ideas for transforming your board, increasing its performance and contributions. Here is a map of where we are headed:

*How can my board transform itself and
the work it does to better fulfill its fiduciary obligations
to our organization's stakeholders?*

Chapter One— Welcome to the Board	*Key questions addressed:*
	• How did the need for governance arise? Why do boards exist?
	• What is distinctive about governing health care organizations?
	• What is my board's overarching obligation?
	• Who are my organization's stakeholders? How do their expectations and interests affect the nature of my board's work?

Chapter Two—
The New Game of
Governance

Key questions addressed:

- How does the environment of my
  organization change?

- How are the forces of change
  reshaping health care?

- What are the implications of these
  changes for governance?

Chapter Three—
Governance
Performance and
Contributions

Key question addressed:

- What factors most influence
  a board's performance and contributions?

Chapter Four—
Governance
Responsibilities

Key questions addressed:

- How should my board focus its limited attention, energy, and time to
  make the most difference and add
  the greatest value? What are its
  responsibilities?

- How should my board fulfill its
  responsibility for formulating the
  organization's ends, its vision, and
  its key goals?

- How should my board fulfill its
  responsibility for ensuring the quality of care?

- How should my board fulfill its
  responsibility for ensuring high levels of executive management performance?

- How should my board fulfill its
  responsibility for enhancing the
  organization's financial health?

Chapter Five— Governance Functioning	*Key questions addressed:*

- What are the roles my board must perform to really govern?

- How can my board formulate policies that effectively guide and direct?

- What type of decisions should my board be making?

- How should my board go about overseeing (monitoring and assessing) the organization's means and ends?

Chapter Six— Governance Structure	*Key questions addressed:*

- How does governance structure influence governance performance and contributions?

- What are the alternatives for structuring governance in health care organizations? What are the assets and liabilities of different structural arrangements?

- What are some ways to get more streamlined governance functioning in a health care organization?

- How should governance work be shared and coordinated between different levels of governance and among different boards?

- What is the right size for my board?

- How many committees should my board have? What types of committees are desirable?

Chapter Seven— Governance Composition	*Key questions addressed:*
	• How should my board go about recruiting, screening, and evaluating potential members? What process and criteria should be employed?
	• How can my board assess the performance of present members before making a decision about renewing their terms?
	• What are the characteristics of the ideally composed board? How can my board move toward this ideal?
	• Should my board have term limits?
	• How should my board remove a disruptive or nonperforming member?
	• How many and what type of ex officio members should my board have?
	• How many physicians should we have on our board? What types of physicians are best for us?
	• To what extent should my board's membership reflect the communities served by our organization?
Chapter Eight— Governance Infrastructure	*Key questions addressed:*
	• How can my board develop objectives, create work plans, and employ agenda and meeting management to enhance its effectiveness and efficiency?
	• How should my board continuously develop its capacities and competencies?

	• How should we evaluate our board, committees, leadership, and members?
Chapter Nine— Board Membership	*Key questions addressed:* • How good a board member am I? • What are the things I should be doing to become a great board member?
Chapter Ten— Transforming Governance	*Key questions addressed:* • How do my board's performance and contributions stack up? • How can my board begin the process of transforming itself?

Throughout the book you will encounter a series of learning and application enablers:

- *Exhibits* that illustrate ideas in instances where a picture really is worth a thousand words.

- A series of *sidebars* designed to supplement the text. They are of three different types:

    Pause and Reflect sidebars like the one a few pages back, offering you an opportunity to focus on your own board. We suggest that you take a moment to think about the questions each one asks and answer them before reading on.

    Illustration sidebars that present examples of key points.

    Perspective sidebars that contain ideas and information that complement the text.

- Twelve *Governance Check-Ups* are strategically positioned throughout the book. They provide you the opportunity to engage in a targeted assessment of your board. To get maximum value from the book, it is

important that you complete these check-ups. They will
be combined in Chapter Ten to produce a map of your
board's overall performance and contributions. Chapter
Nine includes a similar exercise aimed at helping you
assess your own performance as a board member.

• *Benchmark Governance Practices* conclude most chapters, providing a set of high-leverage suggestions for
transforming your board and the work it does.

Board Work is the culmination of our experiences as board members, governance researchers, and governance consultants. We are
deeply indebted to our board member colleagues, research subjects,
and clients for providing us with very different crucibles to develop,
refine, and test our ideas. The health care governance workforce is
small; those consulting and writing in the area can easily fit in most
boardrooms. We've worked with, and learned from, the best—Jeff
Alexander, Barry Bader, Charlie Ewell, Winnie Hageman, Jim Rice,
Mary Totten, Richard Umbdenstock, Larry Wilsey, Roger Witalis, and
Howard Zuckerman, among others. Although we have never worked
with John Carver, his ideas have had a tremendous impact on the way
we think about governance. A special thanks to Linda Miller (president and CEO of the Volunteers of Not-For-Profit Hospitals) for getting us back on track at a critical juncture. We have worked with a
team of gifted professionals at Jossey-Bass; Andrew Pasternack (senior
editor) has been a valued partner from start to finish.

You will have wasted your time if nothing happens as a result of
your reading this book. "Increase the density" of the ideas presented
here—really govern, add value, and make a difference!

March 1999   DENNIS D. POINTER
                                                La Jolla, California
                                                (619)456-1289
                                                JAMES E. (JAMIE) ORLIKOFF
                                                Chicago, Illinois
                                                (312)939-8009

About the Authors

DENNIS D. POINTER has worked with over three hundred clients as a retreat facilitator and consultant. His firm, Dennis D. Pointer & Associates, provides governance development services to health care organizations, nonprofits, and commercial corporations. He is a founding principal of the Governance Advisors of The Governance Institute and a member of the Institute's faculty. He is the author of five other books and over eighty articles; his book, *Really Governing: How Health System and Hospital Boards Can Make More of a Difference*, coauthored with Charles Ewell, won the 1996 American College of Healthcare Executives James A. Hamilton Book of the Year Award. Pointer is John J. Hanlon Professor of Health Services Research and Policy, Graduate School of Public Health, San Diego State University. Prior to joining the SDSU faculty in 1991, he held the Arthur Graham Glasgow Chair of Health Services Management at the Medical College of Virginia. From 1975 to 1986 he was affiliated with the University of California, Los Angeles, where he served as associate director, UCLA Hospitals and Clinics, and professor and chairman, Department of Health Services Management, School of Public Health. While at UCLA, Pointer was a senior research fellow at the RAND Corporation. He is an honorary life member of the Healthcare Forum, a recipient of the Foster G. McGaw Medal of Excellence in Health Administration Education and Research, and has been Dozor Distinguished Visiting Professor of Medical Administration at Ben Gurion University in Beersheba, Israel. He received his Ph.D. from the University of Iowa in hospital and health services administration, and B.Sc. degree in organizational psychology from Iowa State University.

JAMES E. (JAMIE) ORLIKOFF is president of Orlikoff and Associates, Inc., a consulting firm specializing in health care governance and leadership. He was formerly director of the American Hospital Association's Division of Hospital Governance, and director of the Institute on Quality of Care and Patterns of Practice of the AHA's Hospital Research and Educational Trust. Over the last twenty years, he has worked with hundreds of health systems, hospitals, associations, and commercial corporations to strengthen their governance effectiveness, and has served on the boards of several hospitals and civic organizations. He has written eight books and over fifty articles. His books include *The Future of Health Care Governance, Redesigning Boards for a New Era, The Board's Role in Quality Care: A Practical Guide for Hospital Trustees*, and *The Guide to Governance*. Orlikoff is the national adviser on governance and leadership to the American Hospital Association and Health Forum. He is the founding editor and publisher of the *Health Governance Report*, a bimonthly newsletter on leadership issues and trends for health organization board members. He received his M.A. in social and organizational psychology from the University of Chicago and his B.A. from Pitzer College in Claremont, California.

Board Work

1

Welcome to the Board

Symphony boards, professional association boards, school boards, college and university boards, county boards of supervisors, church boards, home owner association boards, commercial corporation boards—in all there are 5.5 million boards in the United States, one for every forty-five citizens! Closer to home, there are approximately 7,500 health system and hospital boards (including those of their subsidiary organizations) and about 120,000 people sit on them.

Some boards meet in plushly carpeted, paneled rooms, with members seated in overstuffed leather chairs around finely polished rosewood tables; everyone is wearing a suit and Mont Blanc pens outnumber Bics. Others convene in conference rooms where members pull up folding chairs to Steelcase tables littered with foam coffee cups left over from the staff meeting that just adjourned.

A diverse lot, to be sure. But beyond these superficial differences, what do they have in common? Why do they exist? Why are they needed? These are important questions that drive to the very heart of governing, regardless of the type of boardroom in which it takes place.

Why Governance?

Boards are late-nineteenth-century inventions. Prior to the mid-1800s most organizations were small, locally focused, and simultaneously owned, directed, and managed by individual entrepreneurs. With the onset of the Industrial Revolution they needed to expand and purchase the facilities and equipment to serve emerging mass markets. Large infusions of capital were required, far beyond the ability of sole proprietors to provide or acquire personally. These funds came from the sale of stock, and stockholders demanded a voice in the affairs of the organizations they now owned. Boards provided the mechanism for stockholder control.

"Going public" led to a division of functions: shareholders owned, boards directed, and managers ran. Lacking the inclination, the expertise, and the time, individual shareholders were incapable of influencing their organizations. Boards, as a special form of corporate representative democracy, were created to protect and advance owner interests. Similarly, management did what boards could not— they ran organizations on a day-to-day basis. Boards became the owners' agents; management became the agents of boards.

Why did boards emerge?	To acquire necessary capital, organizational ownership was transferred from sole proprietors to shareholders. Boards provided the mechanism for the new owners to oversee their investment.
Why do boards exist?	Shareholders are incapable of representing their own interests in organizations.
Why are boards needed?	To serve as shareholder agents, ensuring that organizations function in ways that protect and advance owner interests.

There are some significant differences between the governance of commercial corporations and nonprofits. Commercial corporations have shareholders who own divisible pieces of the organization, be it one share or a hundred thousand. These owners—individuals, mutual funds, trust and pension funds, or other organizations—are easily identified and have similar interests: they all want to maximize the return on their investment. Nonprofits are very different. They have stakeholders, not shareholders, who have a collective and indivisible interest in the organization but do not own it. These stakeholders are often difficult to identify and typically want very different things.

However, for either a commercial or nonprofit board, the overarching obligation is the same: ensuring deployment of the organization's resources in ways that protect and advance the interests of the shareholders and stakeholders.

This is the fundamental *why* of governance. Some important implications flow from this seemingly simple statement:

- *The purpose of a board is to represent and balance shareholder or stakeholder interests.* Standing in for those to whom the organization belongs, boards must decide and act as their constituents would if they had the time, energy, experience, and knowledge to do so on their own behalf.
- *Organizations are means, not ends unto themselves.* In conducting retreats, we often begin by posing these questions: What is your board's central responsibility? Why are you here? Why are you needed? The answers we get follow a common theme: We're here to protect and advance the interests of the organization; its success, its profitability, its growth and development, its market share, its whatever. Answered in this way, a critical point is missed. Organizations are means rather than ends. They are vehicles for achieving shareholder and stakeholder interests. Boards are responsible for ensuring organizations do so effectively and efficiently.
- *Boards are obligated to serve as agents of shareholders or stakeholders as whole.* (In legalese, "as a general class.") Accordingly,

board members breach their fiduciary responsibility if they represent narrow interests or interest groups. Confusion regarding this notion often arises in the case of *ex officio board members*, who hold their seats by virtue of other positions they occupy. Sometimes these board members view their role as representing the specific interests of the group from which they come. Not true. They have the same obligations as other board members: serving as the agents of all stakeholders. There's a difference between how people get to the boardroom door and their obligations once they walk through it.

- *Boards are where the buck stops.* Although ultimately responsible for their organizations, boards are incapable of running them well. As a consequence boards must retain, direct, and oversee professional management. Boards are the owners' agents; management is the board's agent.

- *Boards should have only one direct report, the chief executive officer.* The CEO's task is to manage the organization based on the board's policies and directives. One of a board's key responsibilities is drawing the line between governance and management work; it is a fuzzy one, subject to constant flux as circumstances change. The challenge is providing adequate degrees of freedom so the CEO can do the job creatively while ensuring appropriate direction and oversight. This is a tough balancing act to accomplish, but central to the job of governing. Because of their full-time presence in the organization, specialized expertise, and access to information, CEOs can co-opt or overpower the most dedicated, competent, and hardworking board.

- *Boards can decide and act only through consensus.* Their ability to function depends on their success at weaving together individual talents and perspectives into a reasonably cohesive whole.

- *Finally, boards are part time.* In fact, one of the fascinating characteristics of boards is they exist only for those few hours per month or quarter when they meet—between raps of the gavel. Their only resources (attention, time, and energy) are always in very short supply. As a consequence, to be effective, boards must focus on only those things where they can make the most difference and add the greatest value on behalf of shareholders or stakeholders. This requires tremendous resolve and discipline, as there are a number of things that boards could (and might like to) do that are irrelevant, inconsequential, or better done by others.

Boards come in a variety of different models. Exhibit 1.1 illustrates the ones more commonly found in health care organizations.

Parent boards bear ultimate fiduciary responsibility for the affairs of a corporation, which may have one or more subsidiaries. Although such responsibility may be shared with other boards, the parent retains ultimate authority. Examples are system boards in integrated health care delivery organizations and boards of freestanding hospitals. *Subsidiary boards* are charged with governing organizational components based on responsibilities delegated by the parent board to which they are accountable. The boards of hospitals within a system illustrate this type of arrangement. *Advisory boards* bear no fiduciary responsibility; they provide input, advice, and counsel to management or to a parent board. As a result, the

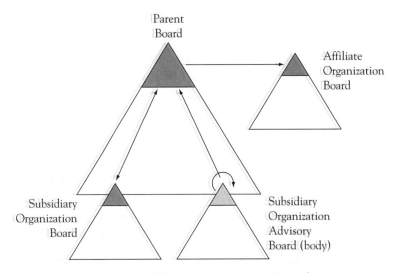

Exhibit 1.1. Types of Health Care Organization Boards

designation *board* is really a misnomer in this case; we prefer the term *advisory body* for them. Many hospitals in investor-owned systems have local "boards" of this type; their functioning is typically consultative, with fiduciary responsibility resting exclusively with the corporate board. *Affiliate organization boards* are governing bodies of separate corporate entities in which an organization has an investment and to which it may appoint or nominate directors.

Governance for Whom?

All boards must answer these four questions to maximize their performance and contributions:

- Why do we exist?

- Whom do we represent?

- What should we be doing?

- How should we go about doing it?

The Why is common to boards of all organizations: representing the interest of shareholders or stakeholders. Next comes Who. The real work of governance begins by answering this question—identifying stakeholders and understanding their interest, expectations, and demands.

Give it a try. *Who are your organization's key stakeholders?* In other words, who depends on your organization and whom does your organization depend upon? Your stakeholders can be either external (customers, purchasers, suppliers, strategic partners) or internal (employee groups). The trick is to identify the most important stakeholders, not every one. Try holding your list to under a dozen. One way to do this is by grouping stakeholders whose interests in your organization and demands on it are roughly similar.

Here are some illustrative stakeholders of a Catholic short-term general hospital:

- The sponsoring religious congregation

- Purchasers and insurers

- Underinsured and uninsured customers

- Medical groups owned by the hospital or tightly affiliated with it

- Physicians and medical groups loosely affiliated with
the hospital

- The community that forms the hospital's primary
service area

Once key stakeholders have been identified, the next step is
understanding what they want and expect from your organization;
those are the interests your board is obligated to represent. Focus
only on the most important demands and expectations of your organization's key stakeholders—the ones that when met (or not met)
have the most significant impact on how stakeholders evaluate the
performance and contributions of your organization. Be specific. It
is helpful to write the statements beginning with the phrases "We
expect" or "We want." Again, give this a try. Pick several stakeholders, put yourself in their shoes, and speculate about their interests and the most important things they want from your
organization.

Here are several key demands and expectations of that Catholic
short-term general hospital's sponsoring religious congregation:

- We expect that all the hospital's clinical programs will
be in conformance with ethical directives of the
Catholic church.

- We expect the hospital's vision, mission, goals, and
strategies to manifest and personify the guiding principles of the religious order that founded it.

- We want the hospital to show a net profit of at least 4.5 percent of adjusted operating revenues. We expect no less than 15 percent of these profits will be employed to provide care to the disadvantaged and underserved, or made available to the benefit trust established by the hospital in this community.

The third step is stakeholder-interest prioritization. What is the relative importance of each stakeholder? What weight and priority should be accorded to their different interests? You can rank order either stakeholders or their specific interests.

Stakeholders are not equal, their interests differ and can even conflict with one another. The question is: Who (which stakeholders), or What (interests), take precedence relative to others as the board chooses among goals, policies, and strategies? This is a critical question that boards must constantly address if they are to be effective. It is impossible to fulfill all stakeholder expectations all the time. If different stakeholder interests are emphasized in different situations, a board will inevitably alienate those it most wants to satisfy. Boards cannot, and should not try to, be everything to everyone. Making consistent decisions based on preestablished prioritizations of stakeholders and their needs is one hallmark of excellent governance.

You have just stepped through a very abbreviated illustration of a stakeholder analysis. If your board were to undertake this for real (and we suggest it does), it would need to do several additional things. First, your entire board, in addition to key management staff and physician leaders, would need to participate in the process. This could be the focus of a one- or two-day retreat. Second, the identification of stakeholders should result from a thorough scan involving the successive generation, elimination, and combination of nominees. Third, the specification of stakeholder interests must be the product of in-depth preparatory investigation (typically undertaken by a board committee with the assistance of management) rather than just speculation. Fourth, given the complexities, a specific methodology would have to be employed to prioritize stakeholders and their interests.

With all these specifics, don't lose sight of the key point: Your board's overarching obligation is *ensuring the organization's resources are deployed in ways that most benefit stakeholders*. To do this, your board must know who these stakeholders are and understand what they want and expect. This is the bedrock of governance.

Here is the first of the series of Governance Check-Ups that you will encounter throughout the book. We strongly encourage you to pause and take a few moments to complete it. Just circle the number that matches your board's approach to each item, then total the circled numbers in the space provided and compare your results to the scoring grid. This will help you engage in a focused self-assessment of your own board in light of the ideas and principles introduced in this chapter. Later on, in Chapter Ten, we'll show you how to combine this check-up with the others to construct an overall map of your board's performance and contributions.

Benchmark Practices: Stakeholders

• Request that management develop dossiers on key stakeholders. Ask for annual reports, newspaper and magazine clippings, press releases, material available through other organizations (chamber of commerce, regional planning bodies, governmental agencies), and special analyses conducted by staff. These dossiers should be summarized and distributed to all board members.

• Invite key stakeholders to your meetings to make brief presentations and engage in a dialogue with the board regarding members' interests, expectations, and demands.

• Hold a stakeholder analysis retreat. We suggest using an experienced governance consultant as a facilitator and devoting at least one day to this activity.

Statement	No	Somewhat	Yes
• My board realizes that its overarching fiduciary obligation is to represent stakeholders and their interests.	1	2	3
• My board understands that our organization is a vehicle (means) for fulfilling the interests of its stakeholders.	1	2	3
• My board has explicitly identified our organization's key stakeholders.	1	2	3
• My board has identified the specific interests, expectations, and demands of key stakeholders.	1	2	3
• My board has prioritized key stakeholders or their interests.	1	2	3

(continued on page 11)

• Constantly remind yourself and your colleagues that the board's overarching obligation is to represent stakeholders and their interests; ensure this obligation is always foreground, never background. If you are the chairperson, make sure a stakeholder orientation permeates all board agenda setting, deliberation, debate, and decision making.

• When deliberating issues, examine them from the perspective of each key stakeholder; "walk in their shoes."

• While a policy is being formulated or a decision made, examine it from the perspective of key stakeholders. Whose interests are being advanced (and to what degree)? To what extent are the demands and expectations of different stakeholders being met? What stakeholder-interest priorities were employed? How would various stakeholders have formulated the policy or made the decision?

Statement	No	Somewhat	Yes
• The vision and goals formulated by my board reflect the interests of key stakeholders.	1	2	3
• My board explicitly takes key stakeholder interests into account when formulating policy and making decisions.	1	2	3
• At least annually, my board formally assesses how well it is representing the interests of key stakeholders.	1	2	3
TOTAL =			

Governance Check-Up: Stakeholders

Source: © Dennis D. Pointer, 1998. Adapted from the Governance Assessment Process (GAP)®. Duplication or use beyond the scope of this book is prohibited.

8	10	12	14	16	18	20	22	24

Low Performance	Moderate Performance	High Performance

• Develop specific plans for constantly staying in touch with key stakeholders. How will you know what they want? How will they know what you're doing?

• Carefully examine key stakeholders and their interests every several years; stakeholders and their interests do change.

• Consider putting representatives of your organization's most important stakeholders on the board or appointing them to the standing committee that deals with vision, mission, and goals; this provides a valuable frame of reference and perspective. However, keep in mind—and constantly remind everyone—that once on the board their obligation is to represent the interests of stakeholders as a whole, not just their own. Most health systems and hospitals already do this. For example, faith-based institutions typically have members of the sponsoring religious community on their boards.

• Each year undertake a formal assessment of how well your board and the organization are fulfilling the expectations and meeting the needs of key stakeholders. Such assessments are difficult to conduct (because they must be customized for each stakeholder), but they are typically worth far more than whatever they may cost to conduct. They go right to the heart and soul of why your board exists, pinpointing its overarching obligations.

The New Game of Governance

Chapter One focused on the why of governance—stakeholders and the role of boards in protecting and advancing their interests. This chapter focuses on the nature of change occurring in the health care industry and its implications for governance. "May you live in interesting times" isn't called a curse for nothing! Health care organization boards certainly do live in interesting—and very challenging—times, primarily because of the change they must contend with every day.

Two Faces of Change

Churches, too!

The health care industry and local markets are undergoing changes across a number of fronts simultaneously. Such changes will have an impact on health care organizations and the ways in which they should be governed. Some will require only relatively minor adjustments, others will lead to significant transformations.

Change occurs in two fundamentally different ways: *Evolutionary change* is gradual and incremental, elaborating and embellishing; the system becomes more of what it already is, like a caterpillar growing longer. Most change we experience is of this type—we get older gradually, not in one-year jumps on our birthday. Organizational performance typically improves or deteriorates smoothly over time, and markets expand or contract like balloons. *Revolutionary*

13

change fundamentally alters the very nature of a system, typically quite suddenly. A whole system is replaced by a totally different one; a metamorphosis occurs, as when that caterpillar turns into a butterfly.

Revolutionary change is less common than evolutionary change, but it occurs a lot more frequently than most people recognize. Evolutionary change builds on and develops what is; revolutionary change wipes out what is and replaces it with something totally different. Evolutionary change modifies the present game's rules; revolutionary change creates a completely new game. Evolutionary change modifies, fills in, and extends the existing *paradigm*—the tacit conceptual framework that defines the way people see their world (Kuhn, 1970; Barker, 1992)—revolutionary change results in a paradigm shift.

Here are a few examples:

Evolutionary Change	*Revolutionary Change*
• Improving the way your business runs	• Starting a totally new business in a different industry
• Growing older	• Dying
• Improving your marriage	• Getting a divorce and marrying someone else
• Developing in your profession	• Changing professions

Not only are the characteristics of evolutionary and revolutionary change different, so are their implications and consequences:

• Forecasting and planning (based on straight-line projections of present and past trends) are very useful during periods of evolutionary change because the future is a direct outgrowth of what already is and was. Such techniques are rendered useless during revolutions because relationships among events and system components arise that cannot be predicted on the basis of trends alone.

• In periods of evolutionary change, systems can adjust slowly. Because the change is incremental, mistakes can be made and penalties will not be all that harsh; evolutionary change is typically quite forgiving. Conversely, revolutionary change demands immediate action, and it is always unforgiving. And when responses are late or wrong, the probability of system failure is very high.

• When change is evolutionary, the knowledge and skills that systems have acquired in the past continue to be useful. The single most important consequence of revolutionary change is that existing system competencies and capacities (the source of past and present successes) depreciate quickly. One of the surest ways of detecting revolutionary change is that it always renders successful systems temporarily incompetent. Think of your own life. You know how to survive and even thrive in a late-twentieth-century urban environment; you know where the danger spots are, how to find food and shelter, how to get care if you're hurt—a whole range of complex knowledge and skills that you've acquired over a lifetime. But say a revolutionary change occurs—you are plucked from your neighborhood and plopped down in the middle of a vast tropical rain forest. How valuable are your urban living skills? They're as keen as they ever were—and they're worthless to you now.

• When change is evolutionary, systems can succeed (even thrive) doing better what they have done well in the past. During revolutions, for systems to thrive (let alone survive), they must do totally new things quickly.

• In times of revolutionary change, systems must learn (quicker and a lot more than in evolutions), but they must first unlearn. Before they can acquire totally new capacities and competencies, they must first jettison all those rendered useless and irrelevant. Significant unlearning always proceeds significant learning. People and organizations are marvelous learners (just watch any infant—

whether human or company). However, we are not very effective and efficient unlearners. It has taken much time and great effort to acquire our present mix of knowledge and skills; we typically do not give them up without a fight.

The Revolution in Health Care

Change always causes misalignment between the incentives posed by the environment and an organization's defining characteristics. In periods of evolutionary change this misalignment is relatively minor, it emerges gradually, and the organization need only make incremental adjustments. However, when the environment undergoes a revolutionary change, a major misalignment occurs—business as usual is no longer possible, and the organization must undertake a major transformation to survive, let alone thrive. A revolutionary change "out there" precipitates and necessitates a revolutionary change by, and inside, the organization.

The financing and provision of health care is undergoing a revolutionary change precipitated by purchasers and customers—who they are, what they are demanding, and how they want to pay. The details are complex and vary from market to market across the country. Exhibit 2.1 portrays an oversimplified summary of the key dynamics.

From the end of World War II through the early 1990s, patients sought services from physicians and hospitals for individual episodes of illness. Patients had insurance policies provided by employers and (after 1966) government covering the cost of their care with no, or very minimal, out-of-pocket expenditures. Because of this coverage, and because they wanted to maximize choice, quality, and convenience, patients were relatively unconcerned about costs. Providers were reimbursed retrospectively based on billed charges or incurred costs for their activity (visits, procedures, days of care); more activity and increased costs produced greater revenues. Essentially, patients entered the health care system armed with checks dated,

Purchasers

Individuals	⟶	Organizations
Little power (dispersed)	⟶	Great power (concentrated)
Cost insensitive	⟶	Price sensitive
Uninformed	⟶	Sophisticated

Demands

Provision of an episodic individual service	⟶	Provision of a comprehensive and integrated service package
Choice, quality, and convenience	⟶	Value

Payment

Retail	⟶	Wholesale
Process	⟶	Outputs and outcomes
Fee for service or costs	⟶	Capitation
Retrospective	⟶	Prospective
The Indemnity Care Game	⟶	The Managed Care Game

Exhibit 2.1. The Revolution in Health Care

signed, and made out to providers. There was only one thing left blank—the amount—and providers filled this in.

Perspectives: Precipitators of a Revolution

In 1965 the United States spent about 5 percent of its GDP on health care; by the early 1990s the figure had grown to approximately 12 percent. Put simply, double-digit yearly growth in the cost of health care was eating employers and government alive—such increases were no longer sustainable. They were seriously harming the global competitiveness of corporations, destroying the budgets of cities, counties, and states, and bankrupting the Medicare Trust Fund. At the same time, purchasers were beginning to question what they were getting for their money. While the United States had the highest per capita health care expenditures in the world, its people were considerably less healthy (as measured by a host of standardized indices) than those of most other industrialized countries. In the minds of most, continuing evolutionary changes in the present health care provision and financing system (or nonsystem) would not solve the problem; more radical—and revolutionary—changes were increasingly advocated.

In the late 1980s and early 1990s a revolutionary change began to occur in the fundamental economic structure and dynamics of the health care industry. Indemnity care was being replaced by managed care. A totally new game with very different rules began to emerge. It was dominated by large, powerful, extremely sophisticated, and very price-sensitive governmental entities and corporations that purchased care for large blocks of beneficiaries. More than anything else, these purchasers wanted to predict and control their health care expenditures and shift financial risk from themselves to insurers and providers of service. For a prospectively set wholesale price per beneficiary, they wanted an integrated and comprehensive array of services that produced specified outputs or predetermined outcomes.

This is a truly revolutionary change. The rules of the existing indemnity care game are not being modified. Rather, a completely new managed care game, with a totally different set of rules, is emerging. There are no more significant changes in the environment of an organization than who its customers are, what they want, and how they pay.

To succeed in this new managed care environment requires "business as *un*usual." Health care organizations must undergo transformations, realigning themselves to totally new incentives. The revolution will be just as gut-wrenching as the ones recently endured by other industries such as banking and air travel. While the specifics will vary from organization to organization, some general patterns are emerging:

- Transformations must be made in all aspects of health care organizations, not just isolated areas. The process will affect their vision and missions, goals, strategies, structure, systems, and key competencies and capacities.

- Vertically, horizontally, and clinically integrated health care organizations—that is, organizations capable of providing a full spectrum of services—are being created. The mechanisms employed in this process include acquisitions, mergers, leases, strategic affiliations, contracts, management agreements, partnerships, and joint ventures (to mention only a few possibilities). The first task entails combining separate organizations. The second is achieving true integration; getting organizational pieces working together in a coordinated and seamless manner.

- Most major metropolitan areas have far more health care facilities and manpower than they need. Because utilization rates are falling precipitously, health care organizations face the incongruous task of significantly downsizing inpatient capacity while simultaneously upsizing such services as ambulatory, long-term, and home care.

Statement	No	Somewhat	Yes
• My board has been slow in responding to significant industry and market changes in the past.	3	2	1
• My board overreacts to significant industry and market changes.	3	2	1
• My board spends at least as much attention, time, and energy envisioning and planning for our organization's future as it does monitoring its present and past.	1	2	3
• My board has a formal method for scanning the environment, industry, and market for changes (both revolutionary and evolutionary) that could have an impact on our organization.	1	2	3
• My board recognizes and deals with evolutionary changes better than it does revolutionary ones.	3	2	1
• My board, management, and medical staff are in sync with respect to how they view the pace and magnitude of change taking place in the industry and market.	1	2	3

(continued on page 21)

- Health care organizations are developing the systems needed to assume and manage the financial risk brought on by managed care.

- Given the economic pressures of managed care, health care organizations are beginning to move from a process to an outcome orientation and significantly redesigning the services they offer and how they provide them.

Statement	No	Somewhat	Yes
• Within the last year, my board has discussed and deliberated the governance implications of changes taking place in the industry, market, and organization.	1	2	3
• My board understands the different characteristics and implications of evolutionary and revolutionary change.	1	2	3
TOTAL =			

Governance Check-Up: Change

Source: © Dennis D. Pointer, 1998. Adapted from the Governance Assessment Process (GAP)®. Duplication or use beyond the scope of this book is prohibited.

8	10	12	14	16	18	20	22	24

Low Performance	Moderate Performance	High Performance

- Health care organizations are shifting their primary focus away from curing specific patients and toward enhancing the health status of populations.

- Health care organizations are forging a wide variety of innovative clinical and economic relationships with physicians.

- Health care organizations are struggling to become far less concentrated on hospital and specialty physician services.

For more on these patterns, see the references listed as Coddington and others, 1994, and Shortell and others, 1990 and 1996. Regardless of the exact configuration health care organizations assume in response to these revolutionary changes, new forms of governance are required. If they are to remain relevant, make a difference, and add value to the organizations they govern, boards must quickly transform themselves and the work they do.

Benchmark Practices: Change

• Help your board keep as foreground the notion that one of its most important tasks is to serve as a guardian of the organization's future on behalf of stakeholders. Most boards spend far too much time analyzing their organization's past and monitoring its present, and far too little envisioning its future. At your next board meeting, take a few moments and look over the last six agendas. What percentage of board attention and time was devoted to "past and present tense" versus "future tense" issues? At least half of each board meeting should be future oriented.

• Spend twenty minutes of each board meeting for a period of six months discussing the most important changes occurring in your organization's environment—describing them and assessing their implications and the specific governance challenges they pose. Each discussion should be preceded by some management staff work devoted to identifying potential changes and framing the issues.

• Dig deeper and learn more about change and its implications. Two of the best books in this area are Joel Barker's *Paradigms: The Business of Discovering the Future* (1993) and Ian Morrison's *The Second Curve: Managing the Velocity of Change* (1996). If you distribute key books like these to board members, the process of transformation will become easier. Boards need a constant infusion of knowledge capital; one of the best sources of new ideas is a targeted reading program designed specifically for your board.

We've been told that the Hopi Indians employ an interesting governance practice. When their leaders meet, two members play the role of the tribe's grandchildren. They are charged with deliberating and debating every issue as their grandchildren might, if present. A very powerful and empowering way of stimulating future-tense thinking!

3

Governance Performance and Contributions

This is the shortest chapter in the book, but one of the most important. Here we raise the bedrock question: What are the factors that most affect governance performance and contributions? We present a model here, then spend the next four chapters exploring its ramifications.

Available research and our own consulting experience suggests that a handful of factors determine how well a board performs and the contributions it makes. The Governance Equation sketched in Exhibit 3.1 identifies these factors and denotes their relationships.

Performance and contributions are outcomes that boards want to maximize. There are two dimensions: effectiveness and efficiency.

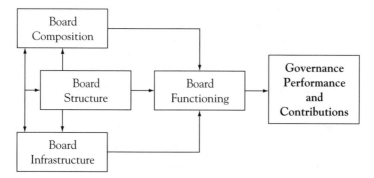

Exhibit 3.1. The Governance Equation
Source: © Dennis D. Pointer, 1998.

Effectiveness is doing the right things and *efficiency* is doing things right. An effective board makes a contribution; it does those things that make the most difference and add the greatest value to fulfilling its overarching obligation: ensuring the deployment of organizational resources in ways that most benefit stakeholders. An efficient board is one that does these things parsimoniously, with the minimum possible expenditure of time, effort, and resources. A board can be effective and not efficient or efficient and not effective—in both instances performance is less than optimal.

Perspective: Governance Research

A very small proportion of the organization and management literature is devoted to governance. If you need some evidence of this, walk through the business section of your local bookstore and count the number of governance titles—if you can find any. We estimate that about 95 percent of this small body of work either describes boards or offers primarily anecdotal prescriptions for improving them. The remaining 5 percent (typically hidden away in academic journals and impossible to understand unless you have recently completed a graduate-level course in multivariate statistics) is scientific. By *scientific,* we mean theoretically based empirical investigations exploring the strength and nature of relationships between board characteristics and their performance and contributions. We have assembled and carefully reviewed every scientific governance study conducted in this century (there aren't that many). Without exception, all of their findings can be incorporated into the governance equation. The descriptive and prescriptive literature has, in our opinion, been hampered by the lack of a valid and widely accepted model of governance; such a model should be employed to describe boards and organize suggestions for improving their performance and contributions. We hope the governance equation is a valuable step in this direction. For those interested in reviews of the health care system and hospital governance literature we suggest the references listed as Alexander (1992), Sofaer and others (1992), and Pointer and Ewell (1994). We are not aware of any comprehensive reviews of the general governance literature.

Board functioning, structure, composition, and infrastructure are independent variables.

- *Functioning* is the variable that has the single greatest impact on performance and contributions. Any adjustment to any of the variables must affect board functioning if it is to do any good at all. If you think of an organization as an organism, this is the physiological aspect of governance: how and how well a board goes about discharging its responsibilities and roles. *Responsibilities* are the things boards must take care of if they are to fulfill their obligations. *Roles* are the activities in which boards must engage. Board members must have a precise, coherent, and shared notion of the type of work they should be doing, and then they must allocate their attention, time, and energy accordingly. Chapters Four and Five explore board responsibilities and roles, respectively.
- *Structure* is the anatomical aspect of governance. It creates the containers for subdividing board work within an organization. Governance structure always depends on—but need not mirror—corporate structure (the way in which managerial and clinical work is organized). Key structural dimensions include board size, number and types of boards, number of governance layers, relationships among boards, and number and type of board committees. The structural aspects of governance are addressed in Chapter Six.
- *Composition* is the raw material of governance; the resources members bring into the boardroom. The primary dimensions of composition include board members' characteristics and their knowledge, skills, and experiences. Boards cannot govern above the ceiling established by their collective competencies and capacities. Board composition is the focus of Chapter Seven.

• *Infrastructure* consists of the systems, processes, and procedures of governance that support the performance of a board's work. Key aspects of governance infrastructure include objectives, work plans, information control, agenda and meeting management, leadership, education and development, and evaluation. Chapter Eight focuses on board infrastructure.

Pause and Reflect: Your Board's Performance and Contributions

Before we begin sharing our ideas for transforming governance performance, take a few moments and think about your board.

• How would you rate your board's overall performance? How does it stack up on effectiveness and efficiency? Regarding the first, how much of a contribution does your board really make—via advancing the interests and meeting the expectations and needs of key stakeholders—to ensuring the success of the organization? Regarding the second, how much time does your board waste dealing with things that don't matter all that much?

• To what extent do you think members have a common assessment of your board's performance? If there are big differences, what might explain them?

• What features of your board (aspects of its functioning, structure, composition, and infrastructure) and the way in which it goes about its work would qualify for the "governance best of breed" award?

• What features most impair the ability of your board to make the difference it should and could?

• If you could make just one change in your board to have the most dramatic impact on its performance, what would it be?

A great board executes those functions—responsibilities and roles—essential for fulfilling its obligations to stakeholders. It is appropriately structured, composed of members who possess the necessary competencies and capacities, and has the needed infrastructure.

Revolutionary changes in the industry and local markets will both precipitate and necessitate equally revolutionary changes in health care organizations, altering their most fundamental characteristics—their vision, strategies, structures, systems, and abilities. To lead this change, governance must undergo an equal transformation in its functioning, structure, composition, and infrastructure. The next five chapters address ways you can help your board accomplish this.

4

Governance Responsibilities

Carver (1991) notes that most boards "are currently performing at a distressingly low percentage of their leadership potential. . . . The problem is not that a group or individual occasionally slips into poor practice, but that intelligent, caring individuals regularly exhibit procedures of governance that are so deeply flawed."

The question is, Why? What separates boards that really govern from those that do not?

Pause and Reflect: A Board Meeting Fairy Tale?

It is 10:05 in the morning on the third Thursday of the month. The chair taps a spoon on her coffee cup and says, "Will the meeting come to order?"

The minutes of the last meeting are approved with a few minor corrections and several announcements are made.

The chair notes that the first agenda item deals with the new ambulatory care center. She invites a partner of the architectural firm retained by the hospital to come in and make a presentation. The architect spreads floor plans and elevation renderings across the table and launches into an overview of the project and the proposed design, inviting board members to ask questions. The board spends the remainder of the meeting happily reviewing and debating every aspect of the proposed design, from the overall site plan to the type of shrubbery that should be planted in the building's atrium. There are a few other agenda items, but no one has the energy to deal with them.

How effectively is this board allocating its precious attention, time, and energy? Is it making a difference and adding value on behalf of the organization's stakeholders? Is it really governing?

An exaggeration? To be sure!! But how often have you witnessed your board commit the sin portrayed in this fairy tale?

A board's performance is most affected by how it chooses to function—a choice over which it has complete control. The most precious and important board resource is its attention, time, and energy. Being part-time entities that exist only when they meet—and meeting for only a few hours each month or quarter—boards have extremely limited amounts of these resources. Therefore:

High-performance boards function in ways that are guided by a clear, coherent, shared, and empowering notion of the type of work they should be doing to fulfill their fiduciary obligations. They focus their limited attention, time, and energy on those things that make the most difference and add the greatest value to protecting and advancing stakeholder interests. Board work is composed of responsibilities and roles.

Responsibilities are things to which board members must attend in order to fulfill their obligations. They are the "what" aspects of governance:

- Formulating their organization's ends, its vision and key goals

- Ensuring high levels of executive management performance

- Ensuring the quality of patient care

- Ensuring their organization's financial health

- Ensuring the board's own effectiveness and efficiency

Roles are sets of activities in which boards must engage to fulfill their responsibilities. They are the "how" aspects of governance:

- Policy formulation—specifying and conveying expectations

- Decision making—choosing among alternatives

- Oversight—monitoring and assessing organizational processes and outcomes

Responsibilities and roles define the very nature of governance, specifying the core functions that boards must perform. This chapter (which focuses on responsibilities) and the next (which focuses on roles) combine to present a complete and detailed map of the type of work a board should be doing.

Ends

An organization has to do something, but can't do everything. Determining what it should do—and what it cannot or will not do—is a board's responsibility. To fulfill its responsibility for ends, a board must formulate the organization's vision, specify its key goals, and ensure that strategies devised by management are likely to accomplish key goals and fulfill the vision. This is the epicenter of governance; a board's other four responsibilities flow from this one. Ends define an organization and provide its identity and direction. Governance is far more about steering than rowing, and the essence of steering is selecting a destination.

Vision

Mention the word *vision*, and what pops into most people's mind is something like this:

East Overshoe General Hospital's vision is to become the market leader and premier provider of acute inpatient care in its service area, offering the highest quality care at the lowest possible cost.

The notion we will be developing bears no resemblance to this meaningless statement.

Perspective: How Vision and Mission Differ

Visions imagine the future, pointing to where an organization should go; missions define the present, describing what an organization is. Visions challenge organizations, missions anchor them. While both are important, we focus exclusively on vision here. After all, a board cannot change where the organization is—that's wholly determined by past decisions. By formulating a vision, however, a board can have a pronounced impact on where the organization should go. Fabricating or refabricating a vision provides a board with its best lever for influencing the organization's future on behalf of its stakeholders.

Visioning entails peering beyond the horizon to that which cannot be seen, only imagined. A vision is an image of an organization's ideal and potentially achievable future state; a definition of what the organization should and could become at its very best. Although they may differ on a number of other attributes, highly successful organizations share one thing in common—a clear, specific, coherent, and empowering vision. The reason is simple: no organization can accomplish what it is unable or unwilling to imagine. Visions spell the difference between purposefully moving and aimlessly wandering into the future.

Although many other groups must be involved in the process, responsibility for formulating a vision rests squarely with the board.

Only it has the authority, as the sole agent of stakeholders, to determine where the organization should head and what it should become.

Visions are vivid dreams, not hallucinations. Accordingly, the formulation must be grounded on an understanding of stakeholder needs and expectations, the structure and dynamics of the health care industry and local market, and the organization's strengths and weaknesses as well as its capacities and competencies. Just as an organization cannot accomplish things it cannot imagine, its board cannot envision things it does not understand.

A vision has two components: core values and core purposes (Collins and Porras, 1996).

Core values are the most important things for which an organization stands. They surface when you picture your organization at its very best and ask the questions:

- What should be the ultimate principles that guide our decisions and actions?

- What should define our organization's heart and soul?

- What should we be most willing to fight for?

- What should we embrace even if it costs us in terms of profitability, market share, or other measures of immediate success?

Illustration of Core Values: Catholic Church–Sponsored Short-Term General Hospital

- Respecting the inherent dignity and worth of all people

- Observing honesty and fairness in our dealings, above all else

- Creating collaborative and mutually empowering relationships with employees and our medical staff

- Infusing the compassion of Jesus into every aspect of the cure and care process

- Being viewed by our communities as an exemplary corporate citizen

- Pursuing operational excellence and fiscal strength with a focus on the long run

---

Values are an organization's constitution, its most central and self-evident truths. Because values must be truly core, we recommend specifying less than a dozen of them.

Core purposes are the most important things an organization strives to achieve. Again based on the organization at its very best, they provide answers to the questions:

- Why should we exist and what should we exist for?

- What benefits and value should we be providing?

- How should we fulfill the interests and meet the needs and expectations of our stakeholders?

Illustration of Core Purposes: Catholic Church–Sponsored Short-Term General Hospital

- Providing, at no out-of-pocket cost, preventive and curative services to the poor or uninsured in our communities that are equal in quality and comprehensiveness to those available to individuals having standard health insurance coverage

- Offering, in partnership with other providers, an array of health care services that are perceived by purchasers to be in the top quartile in terms of value

- Being viewed as the employer of choice in our community; providing employees opportunities for meaningful work and continual development at rates of compensation that exceed the norm

- Funding community organizations, agencies, and programs that prevent disease, promote health, and enhance well-being

---

A purpose is not a listing of products and services provided; rather, it is an organization's reason for being. An organization is chartered by society; purpose (a statement of intended contributions) is the rationale it forwards to society for granting this charter and continuing to reissue it.

Perspective: The Perils of Perfection

In our work with boards, we've discovered an important principle: the desire to do everything perfectly is a formidable barrier to doing anything well.

We'll issue a money-back guarantee: If your board feels that it must come up with perfectly stated core values and purposes, the frustration of not being able to do so will stall and then totally sabotage the visioning process.

Our recommendation: don't shoot for perfection, however defined. Regard everything as a work in progress. Get started, do something, and then continually (and gradually) improve what you have done. Even the illustrative core values and purposes provided in this chapter are far from perfect—but they're still valuable, and the process of improving them would bring its own benefits to the sponsoring organization.

Generating a vision is most often inhibited by the attempt to produce a statement of it. The emphasis becomes wordsmithing rather than substance.

Although the board is ultimately responsible for formulating (or reformulating) the organization's vision, this process
must include others. Initial work is typically done at a one- or
two-day retreat attended by the board, executive team, and
medical leaders. Once a draft vision is prepared, we recommend circulating it widely in and around the organization, and
then holding a series of mini-retreats with key stakeholders,
employee groups, and the medical staff to solicit their input.
During a one day follow-up retreat, the vision can be shaped into
final form.

Key Goals

Visioning, essential as it is, will amount to nothing unless the
board also specifies key goals aimed at fulfilling the vision. These
goals describe a board's most important expectations. The goals
should be:

Few in number, in most instances less than a dozen. Goals
should focus on only the most vision-critical things the board
wants accomplished.

Realistically achievable, but stretching the organization's competencies and capacities.

Quantifiable, providing a precise target and a clear measure of
success, or lack thereof.

Time specific, noting when they should be achieved. This doesn't
need to be soon—the most important goals may take years to
accomplish.

Consistent, so that accomplishing one goal does not impede
progress on others.

Brief, crisply worded, and unequivocal so there can be no confusion about what is expected.

Illustration of Key Goals: Catholic Church–Sponsored Short-Term General Hospital

- Have capitated contracts account for 30 percent of our net profits by 2002

- Have at least 250 physicians in our owned or tightly affiliated medical groups by 2002

- Have our integrated patient care program completely implemented by 2000

- Be ranked in the top decile on HEDIS by 2002

- Have a AA+ bond rating by 2002

- Be allocating at least $250,000 per year to our community benefit trust by 2002

- Have consummated a strategic alliance with a complementary health care system by 2001

A board has an obligation to formulate and convey the most important things it wants and expects the organization to accomplish on behalf of stakeholders. Additionally, strategies (which we turn to next) can only be developed in the context of the targets provided by key goals.

The board—in what must be one of its most important tasks—should assess, formulate, reformulate, and adjust its key goals several months prior to the beginning of each fiscal year. While this responsibility rests ultimately with the board, management and physician leadership must participate in the process.

Strategy

Strategies are plans for deploying organizational resources. To fulfill its responsibility for ends, a board must ensure that strategies

Statement	No	Somewhat	Yes
• My board understands industry and market forces, trends, and developments affecting the financing and provision of health services.	1	2	3
• At least annually, my board is provided with profiles of our . organization's markets and competitors.	1	2	3
• My board understands the needs and expectations of our organization's key stakeholders.	1	2	3
• My board has formulated a clear, precise, and empowering statement of our organization's vision—its core purposes and values.	1	2	3
• My board employs the vision as a frame of reference in its discussions, deliberations, and decision making.	1	2	3

(continued on page 39)

devised by management are likely to accomplish key goals and fulfill the vision.

The development of strategy is a management responsibility. It demands time, technical expertise, in-depth industry and market knowledge, appreciation of competitor strengths and weaknesses, and familiarity with the organization's capacities that go beyond the resources possessed by even the very best boards. Boards should focus on the areas where they can add the most value (formulating vision and key goals), leaving management to attend to those things that it does best (devising strategy).

Here's the process we recommend:

Statement	No	Somewhat	Yes
• Each year my board formulates a set of key goals that must be accomplished by our organization to fulfill the vision.	1	2	3
• Each year my board formally and explicitly reviews, assesses, and approves strategies devised by management to accomplish key goals and fulfill the vision.	1	2	3
• My board has an impact on our organization's ends, specifying its vision, key goals, and strategies.	1	2	3
TOTAL =			

Governance Check-Up: Ends

8	10	12	14	16	18	20	22	24

Low Performance	Moderate Performance	High Performance

1. During the budgetary planning cycle, management develops a set of strategies based on the board's vision and key goals. These strategies would likely be fewer in number and broader than those employed for internal operational purposes.

2. The CEO submits these strategies to the board. Each strategy should be specifically linked to one or more key goals; additionally, an explicit rationale should be provided that explains how the strategy will accomplish the goal to which it is linked, further core purposes, and respect core values.

3. The board then reviews and approves (or rejects) these strategies and, if necessary, management reworks and refines them.

This process respects the distinctive functions and responsibilities of governance and management, subdivides the organization's work effectively, and minimizes potential conflict.

Management Performance

Boards should govern, not manage. A board's responsibility for ensuring high levels of executive management performance flows from this principle. More than any other single individual, the chief executive officer is responsible for the organization's success. Organizations cannot thrive without great management, and they will inevitably fail when it is poor. This assertion is not meant to deprecate the importance of other individuals and groups in the organization, but to drive home an incontestable truth that all boards must face.

The CEO should be the board's only direct report. How a board goes about selecting this individual and developing an ongoing relationship will significantly influence the organization's fate. The board's challenge is to create a context where governance empowers management and management empowers governance. To meet this challenge—and fulfill its responsibility for ensuring high levels of executive management performance—the board must:

- Recruit and select the CEO.
- Specify its expectations of the CEO.
- Appraise the CEO's performance.
- Determine the CEO's compensation and terms of employment.
- Be prepared to terminate the CEO's relationship with the organization, should the need arise.

Recruitment and Selection

Every year approximately 16 percent of health system and hospital CEOs leave their positions; tenure in an organization's top slot averages about six years. These statistics have two implications. First, the office of the CEO comes equipped with a revolving door. Although longevity does not guarantee a CEO will make a contribution to an organization, however, it's nearly impossible for one to do so in a short period of time. An organization with a series of CEO short-timers is at a tremendous strategic and operational disadvantage, for which the board must bear responsibility. Second, the prudent board is prepared when a vacancy occurs. It has a CEO transition plan in place that is updated periodically. We estimate that fewer than 20 percent of health systems and hospitals have such plans.

Illustration: Elements of a Well-Designed CEO Transition Plan

- Who will assume the CEO's duties on an interim basis. (In the vast majority of instances we recommend that the chief operating officer do so.)

- How the present responsibilities of the person who takes over as interim CEO will be shared by other executive management team members. (We recommend that the interim CEO discuss this with the top management team and present a plan to the board within several weeks of assuming the position. It is important that an explicit and precise plan be crafted so the interim CEO does not get set up for failure by the attempt to hold down two jobs.)

- How the interim CEO's compensation will be adjusted to reflect the added responsibilities. (We suggest not increasing the base pay of the interim CEO, as it might have to be reduced later if someone else gets the final appointment. Consider constructing a bonus package; part paid monthly throughout the interim CEO's tenure and part paid in a lump sum at the end of service.)

- If the CEO held a board seat, whether the interim CEO will assume it. (We recommend against this. Rather, the interim CEO should attend all board meetings as a nonmember.)

- Whether the interim CEO will be encouraged, discouraged, or prohibited from applying for the permanent position. (Our advice is to welcome the interim CEO as a candidate. Exclusion might eliminate a potentially attractive candidate or deny the organization the services of a capable interim CEO. An interim CEO who is a candidate for the final appointment should not be involved in the search and selection process, however.)

Note: Adapted from Pointer and Ewell, 1994.

Recruiting and selecting a CEO tests a board's mettle and is one of the toughest and most important decisions it will ever make. Top performers are difficult to find, and the best ones generally are not actively seeking new positions. The process is complex and demands a great deal of board time and energy; other pressing issues must be put on hold, and the organization's metabolism eventually slows down until the process is concluded. The search process requires special expertise, contacts, experience, perspectives, and time boards do not possess. Put bluntly, this is a task that requires professional assistance. Accordingly, the process should begin with the retention of an executive search consultant.

Although each search firm and consultant has its own distinctive approach to designing and conducting engagements, here are some key considerations:

- Appoint an ad hoc search committee composed solely of board members. The committee should be small (fewer than five members) and chaired by the head of the board. The committee should not make critical decisions (for example, choosing a search firm or making the final selection of a CEO) on behalf of the board. Instead, it performs the staff work necessary to optimize the board's time and energy.

- Undertake a comprehensive and in-depth assessment of market challenges; vision, key goals, core strategies, and operations;

the former CEO's strengths and weaknesses; and the past board-CEO relationship.

• Employ these assessments to develop a specification of critical success factors for the CEO. What personal and professional characteristics, experiences, knowledge, skills, competencies and capacities, disposition, and values must the CEO possess to successfully lead the organization into the future and fulfill the board's vision? These critical success factors should be employed by the board, working with the search consultant, to develop a list of candidate screening and selection criteria.

• Throughout the recruitment and selection process do not become distracted; focus on the most important things, including the candidate's record of accomplishment (the single best predictor of future success is past success), whether the candidate possesses the critical success factors and meets the screening and selection criteria, the extent to which the candidate's management values and style mesh with the board's orientation, and the candidate's character.

• Do not evaluate candidates exclusively (or primarily) on the basis of their board interview. Such performances (whether dazzling or disastrous) provide only one view of a candidate in a particular setting at a given point in time. The interview should be just one of many factors employed to make a selection decision.

Expectations

The board exercises influence in and over the organization, on behalf of stakeholders, through the CEO. As the board's only direct report, the CEO is accountable to the board for carrying out its policies and decisions. Accordingly, the board must be explicit and precise about what it wants from and expects of the CEO. Such expectations are the basis on which authority and tasks are delegated to the CEO; they simultaneously differentiate and articulate governance and management work.

Illustration: CEO Performance Expectations

Board expectations of the CEO can either prescribe or prohibit. Typical statements include provisions like these:

- The CEO is prohibited from engaging in, or knowingly allowing employees and agents of the hospital to engage in, any act that would be judged by a reasonable person to be unethical or illegal, or that violates board policy.

- The CEO shall keep the board informed on all important matters affecting the organization's strategic and operational performance, and to deal with the board employing a doctrine of "no surprises."

- The CEO should be involved in the community that constitutes the primary service area of the hospital, as demonstrated by the CEO's being an active member or officer of key community-focused organizations.

- The CEO is expected to behave, in both personal and professional dealings, in a manner that would not embarrass the hospital.

- The CEO is expected to lead a healthy life—physically, psychologically, socially, and spiritually.

- The CEO is expected to attain an average overall confidence rating of not less than 5.0 on the annual medical staff leadership survey.

- The board recognizes and appreciates the stress, workload, and long hours required of the individual who holds the CEO position. As a consequence it allocates generous vacation time to the CEO for relaxation, renewal, and rejuvenation. The board expects the CEO to use vacation time for these purposes. To encourage this, vacation time cannot be accrued nor can it be redeemed for cash compensation if not taken.

- The CEO is prohibited from accepting any gifts or other gratuities that have a value exceeding $50, whether products or services, from individuals or organizations doing or seeking to do business with the hospital.

- The CEO is allowed to engage in separately remunerated activity, including but not limited to consulting engagements and speaking. Such activity must not exceed ten days per year. Its time commitments must be met by taking an unpaid leave of absence (not vacation days), and it must not conflict or appear to conflict with the CEO's obligations to the hospital. The CEO must report to the board chairperson regarding the nature of the engagement and the amount of remuneration prior to accepting an offer.

Clear expectations are essential for building an effective and empowering board-CEO relationship, and are a necessary executive navigational aid. For a board to truly exercise leadership, it must formulate and convey what it expects of the organization's most important and influential employee. We continue to be amazed how few boards engage in this absolutely essential governance practice. Here are some guidelines:

- Specify only the board's most important expectations— the things that are essential for the CEO to do a great job in the eyes of the board as a representative of the organization's stakeholders.

- Incorporate operational descriptions or quantitative benchmarks of performance where possible, but do not avoid stating critical expectations just because they are difficult to measure. Expectations should be subjective (such as the quality of relationships with physicians and the board) as well as objective (those that can be directly measured).

- Focus only on those things (outcomes and means) over which the CEO has a high degree of personal and direct control and influence.

- Involve the CEO in the process. The most meaningful and useful expectations are the result of a dialogue.

- Balance attention between the short, intermediate, and long term. Generate expectations that should be fulfilled by the CEO over varying time frames.

- Update and revise the board's expectations of the CEO at least annually.

- While much of the work should be done in committee, the final specification of CEO expectations should be the result of board deliberation and debate. The board must speak with one voice regarding what it wants.

- Codify the board's expectations. Reducing things to writing encourages precision and provides a foundation for appraising the CEO's performance.

Appraisal

Board members continually evaluate CEO performance; it's unavoidable. The problem is that such assessments are often done only sporadically, conducted within idiosyncratic frames of reference, focused on isolated episodes and behaviors rather than overall patterns of performance, and arrived at without employing explicit, objective, and mutually agreed-upon criteria.

CEO performance appraisal is a governance task essential to ensuring high levels of executive management performance. In addition to working with the CEO as a leadership partner, the board must evaluate the CEO's performance as an employee. Appraisal serves as a bridge between the specification of expectations and determination of compensation. It is one of the board's best CEO guidance and communication opportunities.

While the style and substance of appraisal will vary from organization to organization, the most effective processes share the following features:

- *Focus:* The CEO is the only employee whose performance should be assessed by the board. Although the board might want to be briefed by the CEO on the performance of other key executives, it should never be directly involved in evaluating them. Members of the top management team are accountable to the CEO, not the board.
- *Responsibility:* The process should be conducted and guided by a board committee; this might be the executive committee or an executive assessment and compensation committee. Each year the committee, with board input and approval, should conduct the appraisal in addition to providing feedback to and engaging in performance planning with the CEO. The same committee should be responsible for formulating recommendations forwarded to the full board regarding compensation.
- *Foundation:* Boards experience difficulties designing performance appraisal systems and appraising performance because the necessary prerequisites are not in place. The most critical are a clear vision of what the organization should become at its very best, explicit organizational goals, and precisely expressed CEO performance expectations.
- *Criteria:* The most difficult and challenging aspect of the process is developing appraisal criteria. Although the specifics are idiosyncratic, they should flow from the answers to two questions: First, to what extent did the CEO contribute to the organization's vision being fulfilled, its key goals being accomplished, and its core strategies being effectively pursued? Second, to what extent did the CEO achieve personal performance expectations? That is, the

performance of the CEO should be assessed in light of what matters most.

• *Simplicity:* Performance appraisal can become overwhelmed and eventually rendered useless or inoperable by complexity—of the process, the criteria, the methodology, the forms employed. Keep it simple.

• *Explicitness and candor:* The committee must be prepared and able to provide the CEO with concrete and honest feedback regarding performance. It does no good to pull punches—vagueness devalues the process and does more harm than good. One member of the executive and appraisal-compensation committee should be designated to conduct the feedback session (with other members of the committee present). This person should be someone who is comfortable and skilled in providing explicit, straight, and caring feedback.

• *Action planning:* Appraisal must incorporate planning, answering the question: What specific things must the CEO do to improve future performance? The answer, mutually arrived at by the board committee and CEO, is the ultimate objective of performance appraisal.

Perspective: Why CEO Performance Appraisal Is So Important

• It provides the board an opportunity to better understand the CEO's responsibilities and challenges.

• It is the best mechanism for nurturing and guiding the CEO's development.

• It helps the CEO understand what is important and focus his or her attention accordingly.

• It provides the CEO an opportunity to conduct a self-assessment of performance.

• It helps to clarify mutual expectations: CEO-board and board-CEO.

- It provides the CEO with explicit feedback, direction, and reaffirmation regarding performance.

- It is the framework for developing future CEO performance expectations and goals.

- It is the basis on which the board adjusts the CEO's compensation.

- It fulfills requirements of the Joint Commission on the Accreditation of Healthcare Organizations.

Compensation

The board's clearly stated expectations and its performance appraisal provide the basis for adjusting the CEO's compensation. Because the CEO is its direct report, only the board can make this judgment.

Pause and Reflect on CEO Pay: Do You Know How Much?

We are often amazed by the number of health system and hospital board members who do not know how much their CEO is paid. Many executive and compensation committees believe this to be such a sensitive issue they refuse to inform the board as a whole.

In our judgment, this is ridiculous. As in any nonprofit—that is, 501(c)(3)—organization, the salaries of certain employees are by law a matter of public record. *Anyone,* any reporter, any citizen, any employee, can walk into your business office and request to see IRS form 990, which lists the compensation of the five highest-paid individuals in the organization.

We have seen some board members surprised at their CEO's total compensation package when it was published in the local newspaper. The whole board is the CEO's employer. As a consequence, every member should be aware of the CEO's compensation and the manner in which it is determined.

Although CEO compensation specifics depend on a variety of factors (such as the organization's circumstances and the CEO's own preferences), it must be based on a carefully thought-out, explicitly stated, and clearly articulated philosophy that answers the following questions:

- How is CEO compensation intended to further the organization's vision (core purposes and values) and facilitate accomplishment of key goals?

- At what level, relative to executives in similar institutions, should the board set the CEO's base compensation?

- What proportion of total compensation should be linked to performance? What criteria should be employed to determine the incentive component of the compensation package?

- What should be the terms and conditions of the CEO's severance package?

Here are a few guidelines that your board should consider in managing CEO compensation.

First, this is an arena fraught with sensitivities, complexities, technicalities, and legalities. Accordingly, a compensation consultant should be retained to work with the board and CEO.

Second, CEO compensation should be viewed as a significant investment in the organization's future, not an expense. Value added to the organization by its chief executive should be a huge multiple of the total compensation package. Accordingly, compensation design should be driven by a return on investment perspective where the focus is not on the amount of pay per se, but rather on the value received relative to compensation. This demands that some proportion of the CEO's compensation be directly linked to performance—his or her own and the organization's—and benefits provided to the community. There are a variety of methodologies for doing this, but the board must view its overarching task as designing a compensation package that rewards the CEO for acting in the best interests of stakeholders.

Third, boards must have a clear rationale for the amount of CEO compensation and how it is determined. Internal Revenue Service guidelines for nonprofit institutions prohibit compensation arrangements that amount to private inurement or the distribution of excess revenue that should be used to benefit the community. Compensation judged to be "unreasonable" or "unjustified" can result in civil penalties and may jeopardize an organization's non-profit status.

Fourth, boards must recognize that executive compensation decisions are inherently problematic and sensitive. Some board members may earn only a fraction of the CEO's base salary and never receive a bonus. Compensation considered reasonable by one board member may seem totally out of line to another.

Fifth, specific terms of the compensation arrangement must be codified in an employment contract. What the board expects of the CEO and what it provides if such expectations are met (or exceeded) warrant formalization.

Termination

The CEO's relationship with the organization can be severed for four reasons: death or disability, retirement, the CEO's decision to pursue other opportunities, or forced termination. While the board accepts the first three (often with regret), it must proactively initiate the last. A board's ultimate responsibility for ensuring high levels of executive management performance is defined as much by its willingness to terminate the CEO when the need arises as by its decisions regarding recruitment and selection, expectations specification, performance appraisal, and compensation.

The board must fully and confidently support the CEO. When this is no longer possible and the situation is deemed to be

Statement	No	Somewhat	Yes
• The way in which my board goes about its work empowers and motivates the CEO and top management team.	1	2	3
• Each year my board formulates a set of specific CEO performance expectations.	1	2	3
• Each year my board formally evaluates the CEO's performance employing a set of explicit criteria.	1	2	3
• Each year the CEO is provided with precise, concrete, and candid feedback regarding his or her performance.	1	2	3
• Yearly adjustments in the CEO's compensation are made on the basis of a thorough and explicit evaluation of his or her performance.	1	2	3

(continued on page 53)

irreversible, the CEO must be removed from office quickly. Delay deflects the board's attention, is unfair to the CEO, causes conflict, debilitates the top management team, erodes confidence among the medical staff, and puts the organization on stand-by status.

The CEO should be terminated only for cause. If a CEO exhibits a pattern of disregarding the board's responsibility and authority, repeatedly and consciously violating its expectations and policies, the contract should be terminated. Likewise, if the CEO proves unable to fulfill performance expectations and promote key goals, and the problem does not appear to be correctable in a reasonable period of time, the CEO should not remain in office. With the exception of illegal, unethical, or blatantly imprudent behavior,

Statement	No	Somewhat	Yes
• If the CEO resigned unexpectedly, my board has a plan in place that would ensure smooth interim management transition.	1	2	3
• My board becomes involved in day-to-day operational matters.	3	2	1
• My board makes a contribution to enhancing executive management performance.	1	2	3
TOTAL =			

Governance Check-Up: Management Performance
  Source: © Dennis D. Pointer, 1998. Adapted from the Governance Assessment Process (GAP)®. Duplication or use beyond the scope of this book is prohibited.

8	10	12	14	16	18	20	22	24

Low	Moderate	High
Performance	Performance	Performance

however, a decision to terminate the CEO's contract should never be made on the basis of an individual incident or outcome.

Termination should always be handled with as much dignity as possible. It is important to recognize the CEO's past efforts, accomplishments, and contributions, and to save face for both the organization and the individual concerned.

Quality of Care

Responsibility for quality of output is unique to the boards of organizations that provide health care services. Other nonprofit organizations and commercial corporations can totally delegate this responsibility to management. Because of the presence of a voluntary medical staff (who are typically not employees) and as a result of legislative mandates, court decisions, regulations, and accreditation standards, health system and hospital boards bear ultimate responsibility for ensuring quality. This aspect of governance typically causes board members their greatest concern because of the complexity and mystique of medicine; most directors lack clinical knowledge and experience and find it awkward to pass judgment on the experience, competencies, performance, and care outcomes of individual physicians.

To fulfill this responsibility, a board must:

- Define quality.

- Credential the medical staff.

- Ensure necessary quality and utilization monitoring systems are in place and functioning effectively.

- Employ data generated by such systems to assess the quality of care provided and, when problems are detected, make sure that management and the medical staff undertake corrective action.

This is an area where it is very easy to lose sight of the big picture. Boiled down to the basics, the issue poses three questions that a board must be able to answer: *What is quality? Does our organization provide it? How do we know?*

Defining Quality

Quality is an elusive concept, exceedingly difficult to pin down. However, to fulfill its responsibility for quality, a board must first define it. The reason is simple. If you can't define something, you can't measure it; if you can't measure something, it's impossible for you to improve it.

Illustration: What Is Quality, Anyway?

At a recent meeting a board received two reports regarding the quality of the hospital's rapidly expanding off-site outpatient surgery program.

The first was from the chief of the medical staff, who reported on the results of a detailed and elegant six-month study that conclusively demonstrated that quality, as measured by a series of widely used and valid clinical benchmarks, was superb. The hospital's program ranked in the 95th percentile, or better, across the board when compared with its peer group.

The second report was from the director of marketing, who stated that the program had generated more patient complaints than any other area in the hospital during the past year. She shared a study commissioned to help staff identify and better understand the problem. It was conducted by one of the most reputable consulting firms doing patient satisfaction work, using a questionnaire and methodology validated over five years with hundreds of clients. It showed that patients perceived the program's quality to be terrible (in the lowest quartile) on a host of measures, including scheduling convenience, waiting time, interaction with staff, nurse attentiveness, and the clarity of physician instructions regarding medications and after care.

Quality can be defined in variety of ways:

- Quality is doing the right things, the right way, the first time and every time.
- Quality is exceeding the expectations of purchasers and customers.
- Quality is exceeding established professional norms.
- Quality is the degree to which the process of care increases the probability of desired outcomes and reduces the probability of undesired outcomes, given the present state of medical knowledge.

We intentionally choose not to forward our own definition of quality. This isn't a "cop-out," but rather reflects our strongly held belief that this task must be undertaken by boards themselves.

Exhibit 4.1 presents a model of quality that your board can employ to formulate its own definition.

Quality of care has four dimensions:

Components: quality of the actual content of care (services provided to, and procedures performed on behalf of, the recipient); and quality of the experience as perceived by the recipient

Aspects: quality of the process (activities undertaken); and quality of the outcomes (end results)

Focus: quality as it is perceived by and affects individuals versus a population

Orientation: quality related to enhancing health versus eliminating or minimizing the impact of disease

Each of these dimensions could be incorporated into a board's definition of quality that is realistic, useful, understandable, measurable, and achievable.

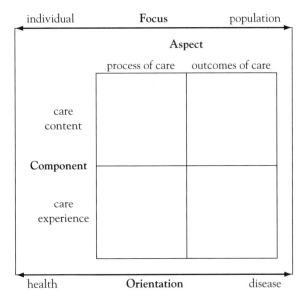

Exhibit 4.1. The Dimensions of Quality

Defining quality provides a framework and foundation for credentialing physicians, ensuring that necessary quality monitoring systems are in place and functioning effectively, and assessing the quality of care provided.

Credentialing

Credentialing is the process that appoints, reappoints, and determines the clinical privileges of physicians (and certain other licensed practitioners). It requires the coordinated activities and actions of many individuals and groups, including the practitioner, the medical staff office, the organization's quality and utilization management department, the medical staff division and department in which the practitioner will be appointed, the medical staff credentials and quality committee, and perhaps also the executive committee, the board quality committee, and the board as a whole. As credentialing is data driven, an information system is needed; the board is responsible for ensuring this system is appropriately designed and functioning effectively. The board must recognize that only it has the authority, on a case-by-case basis, to make decisions regarding which practitioners will be allowed to practice in the institution and what specific privileges they will be granted (the diseases and disorders they can treat and the procedures they are allowed to perform). Medical staff credentialing is the board's single most important quality improvement mechanism.

The major aspects of the process, details of which will vary from institution to institution, are depicted in Exhibit 4.2. Keep in mind that the objective of this process is to assist the board in making two decisions: Who to allow to admit and treat patients (eligibility to practice), and what individual practitioners will be allowed to do (scope of competent practice).

The parameters of the credentialing process have been established over the past twenty-five years through a series of court decisions. These are the basic provisions:

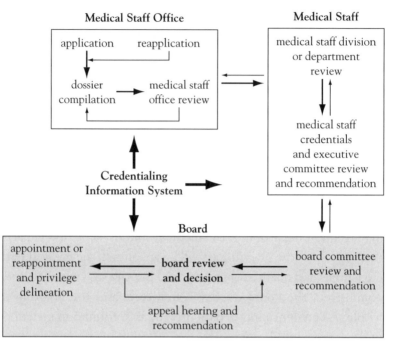

Exhibit 4.2. The Credentialing Process
Source: Adapted from Pointer and Ewell (1994).

- The ultimate responsibility for ensuring quality rests with the board.

- The medical staff is an integral component of the hospital (not separate from it) and directly accountable to the board for the care provided.

- The board is responsible for establishing and maintaining systems and procedures for safeguarding and enhancing the quality of patient care.

- The peer review function can be delegated to the medical staff, but ultimate responsibility for the quality of care must be assumed by the board through its sole authority to grant staff membership and clinical privileges, in addition to its oversight of the quality improvement reporting system.

- The board must exercise a "noted standard of care" in appointing members of the medical staff and maintaining a "system for acquiring knowledge" as part of its "review and supervision" process.

Boards must keep three overarching credentialing principles in mind: First, they alone must make the final appointment, reappointment, and privilege delineation decisions. All steps of the credentialing process preceding board decision making are supportive and advisory, designed to gather and collate information and make recommendations. Second, appointment, reappointment, and privilege delineation decisions must be made by boards on a case-by-case basis after a thorough, careful, and independent review. This review can be conducted by a board committee. The committee then forwards its recommendations to the full board for final approval. Third, boards are responsible for ensuring the effectiveness and fairness of the total credentialing process, not just the steps in which they are directly involved.

Perspective: Top Ten Reasons Why Boards Drop the Credentialing Ball

1. The board believes that its role is to rubber-stamp recommendations forwarded to it, and that the real responsibility for credentialing physicians rests with the medical staff.

2. The medical staff resist board authority in an area they perceive as their own.

3. The board is unfamiliar with the objectives and process of physician assessment and credentialing.

4. Board members do not fully appreciate their legally mandated duties—or their liabilities—in this area.

5. Basic systems and procedures are not in place to help the board assess physician qualifications and clinical outcomes.

6. The board is uncertain of the integrity of the information presented to it, especially dealing with initial medical staff appointments.

7. The criteria employed by medical staff committees as a basis for making credentialing recommendations to the board are vague and subjective, especially in the areas relating to clinical competence, performance, and outcomes.

8. The granting of privileges relies heavily (or exclusively) on the subjective judgments or idiosyncratic criteria of department and division heads.

9. The board receives exactly the same information that the medical staff executive and credentials committee use to formulate recommendations. That is, the board receives primarily raw and unorganized data and has no mechanisms in place to intelligently assess it.

10. Results of the organization's quality and utilization management processes are not meaningfully integrated into appointment and reappointment and privilege delineation process.

A question we get a lot from board members is, "I'm not a physician, so how can I possibly make an intelligent decision about who is a good doctor and who's not?" The answer lies in the proper subdivision of credentialing tasks between the board and medical staff. Simply stated: the medical staff does the heavy lifting—the detailed data gathering—of credentialing, the board ensures that the medical staff has done it right and then makes the final decision.

The medical staff's role is to develop criteria to assess applicants and reapplicants and the specific clinical privileges they want. The staff then applies these criteria fairly, rigorously, and completely in reviewing the qualifications of each individual physician, and makes a recommendation to the board based on the results of this review.

The board's role is to ensure that fair and effective credentialing review processes and criteria are in place, and to compare the results of the criteria-based review for each applicant and reapplicant to the medical staff recommendation. When the criteria and recommendation are consistent, the board approves the medical staff's recommendation (to appoint and reappoint or not appoint and reappoint, and to grant or deny specific privileges). When they appear to be inconsistent, the board requests additional information, sends the application back to the medical staff for further review, or rejects the recommendation.

Systems

To fulfill their responsibility for the quality of care, boards must ensure necessary quality and utilization management systems are in place and functioning effectively; these two systems are complementary and overlapping.

The objective of a *quality management* system is to monitor, assess, and improve the process of providing care and its outcomes. It should answer three questions: Do the clinical practices and processes employed, and the patient outcomes achieved, meet or exceed current professional standards? What initiatives should be undertaken to improve practices and processes and outcomes? What were the results of these initiatives and what should be done to continuously improve quality?

The objective of a *utilization management* system is to monitor, assess, and ensure the efficient use of resources employed in providing care. It focuses on such things as appropriateness of the admissions decisions (both necessity and timing), the length of stay, the level of care provided, the services and procedures performed, the nature and timing of discharge, and the follow-up care provided.

There are two different approaches to designing quality and utilization management systems. The *problem-focused approach* is based on inspection and entails a four-step process:

1. Identifying quality and utilization problems after they have occurred.

2. Investigating and assessing each problem's magnitude, scope, and cause.

3. Initiating action to correct the problem by making changes in systems, procedures, and practices.

4. Monitoring the results and taking follow-up action as necessary.

The *continuous* or *total quality approach* (generally referred to as CQI or TQM), based on the work of Edward Deming (1982), holds that quality cannot be "inspected in" after the fact; rather, it must be "built in" during every step of the process. There are four key aspects to this approach:

1. Understanding the nature of desired outcomes from the perspective of the customer.

2. Identifying and analyzing variations in outcomes.

3. Carefully studying the process (with the assistance of employee teams) to isolate the sources of variations in outcomes.

4. Designing a plan and carrying out a sustained course of action to continuously improve the system so variations are reduced and outcomes are improved.

Health care organizations have typically employed the problem-focused approach in designing quality and utilization management systems. However, spurred by applications in the commercial sector and changes implemented by the Joint Commission on the Accreditation of Healthcare Organizations, health systems and hospitals have been increasingly embracing the TQM and CQI approach. Both are necessary, neither taken alone is sufficient. A good rule of thumb is to begin by devoting a majority of attention on the problem-focused approach. Once it can be clearly, objectively, and conclusively demonstrated that major quality problems have been eliminated or are under control, attention and resources should be gradually shifted to a 75–25 approach over time—75 percent of attention and resources devoted to the continuous approach, 25 percent to identifying and correcting problems.

The board should carefully review the organization's quality and utilization management plans at the beginning of each fiscal year. Questions addressed should include:

- What quality and utilization management objectives (continuing and new) have been specified and how will they contribute to accomplishing the board's key goals and vision?

- How are objectives and systems aligned with the board's definition of quality?

- Are resources adequate for achieving the stated objectives?

- What major activities (for example, reviews, studies, audits, continuous improvement initiatives) will be undertaken during the coming year and what are their objectives?

- What monitoring, assessment, and management systems are in place? Are they adequate? What changes are needed?

- How are quality and utilization management systems integrated and coordinated?

Monitoring and Assessment

Defining quality, credentialing the medical staff, and ensuring effectiveness of quality and utilization management systems culminate in (and provide the means for) the board's direct involvement in assessing the quality of care; the key aspects of which are portrayed in Exhibit 4.3.

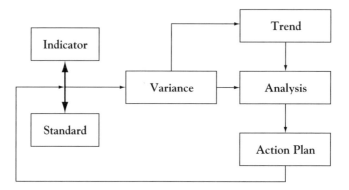

Exhibit 4.3. Assessing the Quality of Care

First, with consultation from the medical staff and management, the board selects a panel of quality and utilization indicators it wants to examine on a continuing basis. These indicators should flow directly from the board's definition of quality. Health care organizations collect an extensive amount of quality and utilization data. The board's challenge is to select a panel of indicators that are representative, comprehensive, quantifiable, valid, and reliable—and, most important, aligned with its definition of quality. There are hundreds of quality and utilization indicators that could be employed; the sidebar provides a small sampling for your consideration.

Illustration: Quality Indicators

- Likelihood that a patient would use the organization's service again (experiential process and outcomes of care indicator)

- Severity-adjusted average length of stay and total cost per discharge for the top ten diagnosis-related groups or service lines (process- and outcome-oriented indicator)

- Hospital-acquired-infection rate (content-oriented outcome indicator)

- Percentage of newborn babies weighing less than 2,500 grams (content-oriented outcome indicator)

- Rate of unplanned admissions following an ambulatory surgery procedure (content-oriented process indicator)

- Employee and medical staff satisfaction (process-oriented indicator)

- Proportion of individuals in the service area who engage in some form of strenuous exercise at least two times per week (population-based, health-focused process indicator)

- Smoking rate in the service area (disease-focused population indicator)

- Medication error rate (process-oriented content indicator)

Second, for each indicator a standard is specified—a level the indicator should either approach, not exceed, or fall below. Standards can be obtained from a variety of different sources: published norms, the organization's own past performance, and data collected by federal and state agencies, hospital associations, commercial vendors, and the Joint Commission on the Accreditation of Healthcare Organizations.

Third, trends in the variances between indicators and standards are portrayed and their causes and sources analyzed using a problem-focused or continuous approach.

Fourth, on the basis of its review and assessment, the board requests management or medical staff to submit plans of action to correct the deficiencies or to continuously improve the underlying processes in such a way that quality is enhanced.

Much of the work entailed in this process is, of course, performed by management and the medical staff. However it is critical that the board be directly involved in selecting indicators, analyzing variances and trends (we suggest at least once per quarter), and reviewing quality enhancement action plans and their results.

Statement	No	Somewhat	Yes
• My board has formulated a comprehensive and rigorous definition of quality.	1	2	3
• Based on recommendations forwarded by the medical staff, our board (board committee or in a system, subsidiary board) thoroughly evaluates the experience, competence, performance, and outcomes of each individual physician prior to appointment or reappointment to the medical staff and determination of clinical privileges.	1	2	3
• My board periodically assesses the rigor, thoroughness, objectivity, and fairness of the credentialing process, in addition to its conformance with the requirements of the law, applicable regulations, and JCAHO standards.	1	2	3
• My board makes sure that our organization has the necessary quality and utilization management systems in place and functioning effectively.	1	2	3

(continued on page 67)

Statement	No	Somewhat	Yes
• My board has formulated a set of explicit standards that convey its expectations regarding the quality of care provided by and in our organization.	1	2	3
• Employing a set of specific quantitative indicators, my board periodically monitors and assesses the quality of care provided in and by our organization.	1	2	3
• When monitoring and assessment of the quality of care indicates there are problems, my board has a mechanism in place to ensure that corrective action is undertaken.	1	2	3
• My board makes a contribution to enhancing the quality of care.	1	2	3
TOTAL =			

Governance Check-Up: Quality

Source: © Dennis D. Pointer, 1998. Adapted from the Governance Assessment Process (GAP)®. Duplication or use beyond the scope of this book is prohibited.

8	10	12	14	16	18	20	22	24

Low
Performance

Moderate
Performance

High
Performance

Finances

The financial challenges facing health care organizations now are of far greater magnitude and a very different type than in the past. To meet these challenges and fulfill their responsibilities for ensuring the organization's financial health, boards must:

- Specify financial objectives.

- Make sure plans and budgets developed by management are aligned with and promote achievement of financial objectives, key goals, and the board's vision.

- Monitor and assess financial performance and, when problems are detected, ensure corrective actions are undertaken by management.

- Ensure that necessary financial controls are in place.

Health care organizations must generate sufficient revenues and manage expenses and produce margins, and must do so in a manner that protects and advances stakeholder interests. The board's responsibility for finances stems from this reality.

Objectives

The board's protection of the organization's financial health begins with the specification of clear and precise financial objectives, as illustrated in Exhibit 4.4.

Financial objectives must flow from the board-formulated vision and key goals. They serve as a foundation for financial planning, performance monitoring and assessment, and the establishment of necessary controls.

Financial objectives must answer three questions: What is the board's definition of financial health? What must the organization achieve financially to accomplish key goals and fulfill the vision? How should financial performance be assessed?

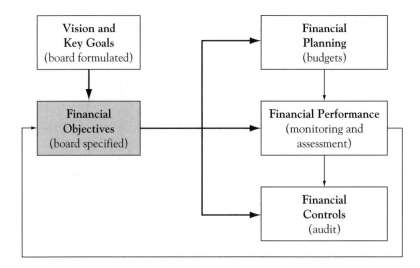

Exhibit 4.4. Assuming Responsibility for Finances

Each year the board, assisted by its finance committee and with input and counsel from the CEO and chief financial officer, should draft a set of financial objectives. Such objectives should be comprehensive, covering all areas of financial performance and health; specifically linked to key goals; and directly related to fulfilling the vision. The objectives must be quantifiable so the board can assess the extent to which they have been accomplished.

Illustration: Financial Objectives

The board expects:

- The organization will achieve an overall net profit from operations of X.X percent of gross operating revenue.

- Operating revenues will grow at the rate of not less than X percent per year.

- A third-generation cost accounting system will be installed and operable by the third quarter of next year.

- The organization will achieve a return on equity of not less than XX percent.

- Total EBITDA [earnings before interest, taxes, depreciation, and amortization] from all for-profit subsidiaries will increase by at least X percent during the next five years.

- Severity-adjusted cost per inpatient discharge will be reduced by XX percent over the next three years.

- Net yield on investment income (adjusted for inflation) will be at least X.X percent.

Financial objectives should be formulated by the board in at least five areas:

Bottom line: Quarterly and year-end operating and nonoperating margins for the organization as a whole and major lines of business

Cash: Amount of cash on hand by quarter and at year end

Operations: Relative priority that should be given to various categories of programs and services (both ongoing and new)

Capital: Relative priority that should be given to different programmatic categories of investment in plant and equipment

Performance: Targets established for an array of ratios that measure specific aspects of financial performance

Clear, precise financial objectives, linked to vision and goals, state what the board expects. They provide management with a framework and specific guidelines for developing financial plans.

Planning and Budgets

Boards do not have the time, experience, or expertise to engage in financial planning; this is a task that must be delegated to manage-

ment (the same argument we make regarding the board's involvement in strategic planning). However, to fulfill its responsibility, the
board must ensure that management's plan protects and advances
stakeholder interests by achieving board-specified financial objectives, key goals, and vision.

Perspective: Types of Budgets

An *operating budget* forecasts the revenues generated from, and the
expenses incurred by, engaging in key organizational activities. It con-
solidates detailed financial plans prepared for the organization as a
whole and for individual lines of business, departments, divisions, and
programs.

A *cash budget* forecasts the sources and uses of cash. It projects quarterly beginning and ending cash receipts, disbursements,
and balances by major category.

A *capital budget* details planned expenditures for additions, modifications, and renovations to plant, and the purchase or lease of new
equipment. Funds for capital investment come from depreciation,
operating margins, gifts, and investment income.

The financial planning process culminates in the preparation of
budgets, of which there are three types: operating, cash, and capital. Boards are often required to review and approve these budgets.
Overwhelmed by their weight, detail, and complexity, and the massive effort that went into preparing them, this task is usually cere-
monial. How then does the board exercise appropriate influence on
behalf of stakeholders in this process? Here are some suggestions:

•   First, budgets should be thought of as management's plans
for allocating resources to achieve board-formulated financial
objectives (in addition to key goals and vision). Budgets are means

proposed by management to achieve what the board wants and expects. This is an obvious principle, but one that often gets lost in the shuffle. It is critically important to keep it in the foreground.

- The types of budgets management needs to run organizations are quite different from the ones boards require to govern them. Management, with direction and input from the board's finance committee, should be requested to prepare governance-friendly and focused operational, cash, and capital budgets for board review. These budgets should be composed of highly aggregated categories that reflect board-formulated financial objectives.

- Management should be requested to file a memorandum with the budget describing to the board how each category facilitates fulfilling the vision, accomplishing key goals, and achieving financial objectives.

- The governance-focused budget and memorandum should be carefully analyzed (and if necessary sent back to management to be reworked) by the board's finance committee prior to being forwarded to the board for review.

- Contrary to prevailing practice, we recommend the board not approve the budget (unless required to do so by law), but rather pass a resolution stating it is aligned with vision, key goals, and financial objectives. Budgets are management tools, albeit ones that have significant governance implications. Boards should focus on financial objectives and the extent to which budgets lead to their accomplishment, and should stay out of budget detail.

Assessment

Financial plans are promises made to the board by management. To fulfill its responsibility for the organization's financial health, the board must make sure such promises are fulfilled. It does so—as sketched in Exhibit 4.5—by monitoring and assessing financial per-

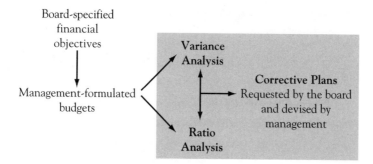

Exhibit 4.5. The Financial Monitoring and Assessment Process

formance as reflected in the revenue and expense statement, cash flow statement, and balance sheet.

The two techniques the board uses to monitor financial performance are variance analysis and ratio analysis. *Variance analysis* compares budget projections with results, addressing these questions: What was promised? What actually happened? What is the nature, magnitude, and consequences of the differences? *Ratio analysis* examines specific statistics designed to quantify an organization's financial status.

Illustration: Financial Ratios

A variety of financial ratios have been developed. The most widely employed fall into these four categories:

Liquidity ratios measure an organization's ability to meet short-term obligations. For example:

- Current ratio: current assets ÷ current liabilities

- Acid test ratio: (cash + marketable securities) ÷ current liabilities

Activity ratios measure the ability of different types of assets to generate net operating revenue. For example:

- Total assets turnover ratio: total operating revenue ÷ total assets

- Cash turnover ratio: net operating revenue ÷ (cash + marketable securities)

Capital structure ratios measure the organization's ability to meet long-term obligations. For example:

- Debt service coverage ratio: (net income + depreciation) ÷ (debt principal payment + interest)

- Average age of plant ratio: accumulated depreciation ÷ depreciation expense

Profitability ratios measure the organization's ability to generate margins from operations. For example:

- Return on assets ratio: net income ÷ total assets

- Operating margin ratio: (operating revenue – operating expense) ÷ operating revenue

---

In assessing financial performance, the same process should be employed as we suggested for quality of care.

- A panel of indicators (variance measures and financial ratios) are selected by the board with management assistance. The indicators should reflect board-formulated financial objectives and be drawn from all key financial statements. They must be the most important ones—the ones that best reflect the organization's financial health, or lack thereof. We recommend selecting fewer than twenty indicators.

- Standards (percentage of acceptable variance and financial ratio targets) are developed for all indicators.

- The board's finance committee and the full board review the panel of indicators and compare them to established standards at least quarterly.

- When analysis indicates unacceptable performance, the board requests that management prepare a plan to correct the problem.

Controls

To fulfill its responsibility for finances, the board must make sure that accounting systems for supplying accurate and timely information are in place and functioning effectively; that transactions are properly authorized, executed, and recorded; and that financial statements reflect current financial status. This is accomplished through an annual audit performed on behalf of the board by a certified public accounting firm that examines the organization's financial statements; ascertains if procedures and practices are in accordance with generally accepted accounting principles; assesses the adequacy of financial, accounting, and control systems; and forwards recommendations to the board and management regarding modifications and improvements.

To safeguard the organization's assets and see to it they are used for legitimate purposes in legitimate ways, the board (with the assistance of its audit committee) must:

- Appoint or reappoint the external auditor and approve the audit's scope and approach and associated fees.

- Review the auditor's formal opinion and management letter, which presents conclusions regarding the organization's financial condition and recommendations for alterations in systems, procedures, and practices.

- Require management to devise and execute plans to correct any deficiencies.

- Ensure that the organization's internal audit function is properly structured and effective.

Statement	No	Somewhat	Yes
• Members of my board have the knowledge necessary to understand, interpret, and evaluate our organization's financial statements.	1	2	3
• Each year my board formulates a set of explicit financial objectives for our organization.	1	2	3
• My board ensures that financial objectives are aligned with our organization's key goals and vision.	1	2	3
• At least annually, my board reviews management plans and budgets, and assesses whether we are likely to accomplish specified financial objectives.	1	2	3
• Employing specific quantitative measures (such as variances and financial ratios), my board periodically monitors and assesses our organization's financial performance.	1	2	3
• When monitoring and assessment of financial performance indicates there are problems, my board has a mechanism in place to ensure corrective action is undertaken.	1	2	3

(*continued on page 77*)

Governance Responsibilities   77

Statement	No	Somewhat	Yes
• Each year my board meets with the external auditors, reviews their opinions, and ensures that management makes and executes plans to correct any deficiencies.	1	2	3
• My board makes a contribution to enhancing our organization's financial health.	1	2	3
TOTAL =			

Governance Check-Up: Finances
   Source: © Dennis D. Pointer, 1998. Adapted from the Governance Assessment Process (GAP)®. Duplication or use beyond the scope of this book is prohibited.

8	10	12	14	16	18	20	22	24

Low   Moderate   High
Performance   Performance   Performance

Self-Management

Boards are responsible for governing their organizations, but to do so they must first govern themselves. To assume responsibility for itself a board must make sure the following conditions are met:

- Its structure effectively subdivides and coordinates governance responsibilities, roles, and tasks within the organization.

- Its composition provides the competencies and capacities needed to govern.

- Its infrastructure (systems and procedures) supports the performance of governance work.

Board structure is the focus of Chapter Six. Board composition will be addressed in Chapter Seven, and infrastructure in Chapter Eight.

Benchmark Practices: Responsibilities

• Once stakeholders and their interests are identified and thoroughly understood, a board must develop a clear, precise, coherent, shared, and empowering definition of the responsibilities it must fulfill to shape and lead the organization. What are the most important things your board should be doing to protect and advance stakeholder interests? In this chapter we have forwarded our answer to this question; we commend these notions to you. *But* achieving consensus regarding responsibilities is a task your board must undertake for itself—no one else's ideas will serve you well. Accordingly, we urge your board to carve out a block of time to explicitly consider, talk through, deliberate, debate, and arrive at consensus regarding its responsibilities.

• Before your board can begin focusing on those things that matter most—its responsibilities—it must undertake a governance housecleaning. To free up attention, time, and energy for assuming and fulfilling its responsibilities, your board must first stop doing things that are inconsequential, irrelevant, or better done by others (management and medical staff). Conduct an audit of every agenda item addressed in your last half-dozen meetings, assessing the extent to which your board is focusing on those issues that matter most. On the basis of this audit: What items and issues could and should have been totally eliminated from the board's agenda, or the amount of time devoted to them significantly reduced? Begin employing your board's specification of its responsibilities as a screening and guidance tool to decide what issues and items get on the agenda (with few exceptions, only those directly related to the board's responsibilities) and how much time should be devoted to them (depending their criticality and significance to vision and key goals).

- Review results of the four governance check-ups you have completed in this chapter. Focus your board's attention on those areas of responsibility where its functioning is problematic. Here are some questions to get you started:

If you scored low on the ends check-up:

How can your board formulate and reformulate an empowering vision for the organization that reflects its core purposes and values?

What are the key goals that must be accomplished to fulfill the vision?

What should you do to ensure that strategies devised by management are aligned with—and likely to achieve—key goals and the vision?

If you scored low on the management check-up:

How will you ensure that if a vacancy arises in the chief executive officer position, the transition and the recruitment and selection process will be smooth and successful?

How can your board specify and convey its most important expectations of the CEO?

How should you appraise the CEO's performance?

How should you determine the CEO's compensation?

What preparations do you need in order to be able to terminate the CEO if the need arises?

If you scored low on the quality check-up:

How can your board define what it means by quality, taking into account the concept's multifaceted nature?

What procedures should you establish for appointing, reappointing, and determining privileges of the medical staff?

How can you ensure necessary quality monitoring systems are in place and functioning effectively?

How can you best employ data generated by such systems to evaluate the quality of care and, when problems are detected, ensure corrective action is undertaken by management and medical staff?

If you scored low on the finances check-up:

What should you do to specify financial objectives?

How can you ensure plans and budgets developed by management are aligned with, and lead to the achievement of, your financial objectives, key goals, and vision?

How can you monitor and assess financial performance and, when problems are detected, ensure corrective action is undertaken by management?

What should you do to ensure that necessary financial controls are in place?

For each of the ideas that you (or better yet, your full board) have generated, develop an action plan:

What specifically must be done to improve your board's performance?

How will it be undertaken? List the specific steps that must be executed.

Who will be responsible? A standing or ad hoc committee of the board? Note the input and assistance required from management, the medical staff, and (possibly) consultants.

When will it be accomplished?

5

Governance Functioning

Responsibilities and roles are complementary aspects of governance functioning. Responsibilities are the *what* of governance (the things that require boards' attention); roles are the *how* (the things they need to do). This chapter focuses on the three roles all boards must execute to maximize their performance and contributions:

- Policy formulation—conveying expectations and directives

- Decision making—choosing among alternatives

- Oversight—monitoring and assessing organizational processes and outcomes

Policy Formulation

When asked if matters of policy are important and the things on which they should be spending a good bit of their time, board members typically answer with a resounding yes. But when we ask them to show us their policies, we typically get blank stares, assertions like "we have 'em but they're in our minutes," or photocopies of the by-laws (policies to be sure, but dealing only with the board's responsibility for itself). While all boards recognize the importance of policy, few of them do much with it in practice.

Perspective: Policy Governance

Our ideas about the board's policy formulation role have been influenced by the work of John Carver. For those desiring a more in-depth treatment of policy as the cornerstone of governance, we strongly recommend his *Boards That Make a Difference* and (with Miriam Mayhew Carver) *Reinventing Your Board: A Step-by-Step Guide to Implementing Policy Governance* and *CarverGuide 1: Basic Principles of Policy Governance,* all from Jossey-Bass. To order, call 800–956–7739.

The single most important board role is policy formulation; it is the primary mechanism boards have to influence their organizations and it provides the best tangible evidence that responsibilities are being fulfilled on behalf of stakeholders. Additionally, execution of the decision-making and oversight roles depends on a comprehensive set of well-formulated policies. To truly make a difference, the center of governance work must be policy formulation.

A *policy* is a statement of intent that guides and constrains subsequent decision making and action, as well as the delegation of authority and tasks (adapted from Carver, 1991).

To employ policy as a leadership tool, boards must:

- Agree on the functions and focus of policy, why policies are needed and what they should be formulated about.

- Agree on the form of a policy, whether to prescribe or prohibit specific ends or means.

- Determine the specificity of a policy, the degree to which it directs and constrains.

Functions and Focus

It is through formulating policy that boards exercise voice in organizations. Policies perform two absolutely essential functions. First, they express board expectations—of the organization as a whole, of itself, of management and the medical staff. Policies are the means by which boards specify and convey what they want done (and what they want the organization to refrain from doing) in addition to the range of acceptable (and unacceptable) means for accomplishing specified goals. To lead rather than follow, policies must clarify and articulate board expectations. Second, policy is the mechanism by which boards direct and constrain as they delegate authority and tasks to management and the medical staff.

Board policies shape the way in which management and the medical staff undertake their work. As illustrated in Exhibit 5.1, board policies are at the very top of a pyramid; they are an organization's most important pronouncements. From them flow management and medical staff operating policies, procedures, and rules, and the individual decisions and actions that constitute an organization's real work. Boards exercise influence and leverage not by focusing on the specifics (there are just too many of them), but rather by framing and crafting the context in which action takes place.

What can boards formulate policy about? The answer, of course, is anything they choose (as far as applicable laws permit). However, to make the most difference and add the greatest value—given their extremely limited attention, time, and energy—boards must formulate policy only about their most important responsibilities.

A board fulfills its responsibility for ends by formulating policies regarding:

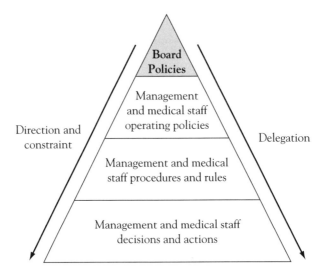

Exhibit 5.1. The Policy Pyramid

- Key stakeholders—who they are and what they need and want

- Vision—the organization's core purposes and core values

- Key goals—what must be done to fulfill the vision

- Strategic oversight—the nature of management's task of devising strategy

- Linkage—between management strategies and board-formulated vision and goals

A board fulfills its responsibility for ensuring high levels of executive management performance by formulating policies regarding:

- Succession—the way a transition should be handled when the CEO position becomes vacant, including recruitment and selection processes

- Standards—expectations for CEO performance critical to carrying out the organization's mission and meeting its goals

- Methodology—the procedures and criteria employed to assess the CEO's performance

- Incentives—the way in which the CEO's compensation is determined

- Defensive action—conditions causing a decision to terminate the CEO and the way it would be done

A board fulfills its responsibility for ensuring the quality of care by formulating responsibilities regarding:

- Definition—what constitutes quality for this organization

- Staff selection—the process and criteria for appointing, reappointing, and determining privileges of the medical staff

- Information infrastructure—the way in which quality and utilization systems should be built and how they should function

- Monitoring—the process and criteria employed to track and assess the quality of care

A board fulfills its responsibility for ensuring the organization's financial health by formulating policies regarding:

- Financial objectives—critical milestones for accomplishing key goals and fulfilling the vision

- Budget specifications—the nature of management's task of devising financial plans (budgets)

- Budget oversight—the alignment of management-devised budgets and board-formulated financial objectives, key goals, and vision

- Financial review—the processes and criteria employed to assess the organization's financial performance

- Financial controls—the kinds of procedures that must be in place to protect the organization

A board fulfills its responsibility for self-management by formulating policies regarding:

- Governance structure—how board work will be subdivided and coordinated

- Governance composition—specification of needed board member competencies and capacities

- Governance infrastructure—systems and procedures that must be in place to support performance of the board's work

Employing this responsibilities framework, boards must pursue their own policy agenda. Stakeholder interests and organizational circumstances are unique, and so too must be the board's expectations and directives and the policies it formulates regarding them. This is not an arena where a board should adopt (or adapt and rewrite) off-the-shelf model policies developed by others. Although Appendix A offers samples of board policies for each responsibility area, the policies listed there are designed only to demonstrate the kinds of things to consider. We suggest that you peruse these illustrative policies before proceeding, and then set them aside and go on to review your own policy requirements based on your own situation.

Form

Board policies come in many different shapes and sizes. A board can choose to convey expectations by being prescriptive, stating its "thou shalts," or by being prohibitive, articulating "thou shalt nots" that limit and restrict. Additionally, board policies can deal with either organizational *ends* (vision, key goals, and the linkage between strategy, vision, and goals) or *means* (executive performance, quality of care, finances, and self-management).

As illustrated in Exhibit 5.2, there are four different forms of board policy:

Prescribing ends: For example, specifying the organization's vision and key goals.

Prescribing means: For example, directing that a particular program be undertaken.

Prohibiting ends: For example, stating that certain populations should not be served or a specific program should not be initiated.

Prohibiting means: For example, barring investment of the organization's excess funds in certain types of financial instruments.

Boards convey what they want and expect by prohibiting and prescribing organizational ends and means. However, we have found the most effective policies prescribe ends and prohibit means.

Ends are destinations a board wants the organization to move toward and arrive at. The most effective way of conveying expectations about ends is by simply designating them; the board says "head that-a-way" or "accomplish this." The prescribed end then serves as a beacon, drawing the organization onward.

	Ends	Means
Prescriptions	**Policies that prescribe certain ends**	Policies that prescribe certain means
Prohibitions	Policies that prohibit certain ends	**Policies that prohibit certain means**

Exhibit 5.2. Forms of Board Policy

Means—ways of reaching a prescribed destination—should not be prescribed. It is tempting to direct an organization to use certain means in pursuing its ends, but in the vast majority of instances, this is a serious error. There is no limit to the number of means that can be prescribed, so the board will soon get bogged down in details if it tries this approach. Also, directing how to do something automatically eliminates all other alternatives, and there may well be better ways than the ones that come to mind first. Furthermore, designating means brings a board dangerously near—if not across—the line that separates governing an organization from running it.

Instead, boards must convey their expectations about important means. In doing so, we suggest they prohibit, limit, and restrict rather than prescribe. Given the almost infinite array of potential (and feasible) means, many of which cannot be imagined ahead of time, it is far more effective and efficient for a board to specify those that are not acceptable. As Carver (1997) observes: "At first glance, this sounds a little odd and rather negative because the board deals with means by producing a 'don't do list.' Ironically, this verbally negative language is psychologically positive because it allows a freedom, the boundaries of which need not be guessed. This action by the board is like building an enclosure within which freedom, creativity, and action are allowed and even encouraged."

Specificity

By formulating policy boards convey expectations and delegate tasks in their areas of responsibility by prohibiting and prescribing ends and means. The remaining question, and the one that typically causes boards some of their greatest policy formulation difficulties, is, How specific and directive does a board need and want to be? The answer determines the extent to which a board exercises influence on behalf of stakeholders and where it establishes the dividing line between governance and operations. Consider the extremes. If a board formulates only a few very broad policies it abdicates its responsibilities; the board either has no expectations or is unable and unwilling to convey them, and is not really governing. If, on the other hand, it formulates a mountain of extremely detailed policies telling management and the medical staff what to do, and not do, in every conceivable situation, the board is running—not governing—the organization.

Board policies can range from the very broad, allowing considerable latitude, to the quite specific, allowing only narrow degrees of freedom and discretion. So how specific should a board be? Based on the work of Carver (1991, 1996, 1997) we offer a principle:

A board should formulate a policy with enough specificity that it is willing to accept any reasonable interpretation, application, or implementation of it.

A board exercises influence in and over an organization by conveying expectations and directing delegated tasks so organizational resources are deployed in ways that protect and advance shareholder interests. Each time a policy is formulated, a board must ask, What degree of specificity is necessary to ensure these expectations are interpreted appropriately and the delegated task will be executed in the manner intended? Our answer: continue to increase the specificity of a policy until a point is reached where the board is willing to accept any reasonable interpretation, application, or effort to implement it. This defines the point which the board hands off its policy (to its own committees or to management or the medical staff), comfortable that an appropriate level of accountability is ensured.

The potential specificity of a policy is like boxes of different sizes that can be placed inside one another. As a board feels the need to be more explicit about its expectations and allow fewer degrees of freedom when delegating a task, it constructs a smaller box. The size of the box defines where the board's intent ends and all subsequent decision making and action commences. The board is saying, essentially, "If you respect our directives and limits (that is, stay within the box) and make a reasonable effort to comply, we will accept whatever you do."

The specificity and associated accountability a board needs to be comfortable is affected by four factors:

- *Trust and experience:* Trust is a result of the extent to which past commitments have been fulfilled. Where commitments have been met over a long period of time, trust is high; when they have not been fulfilled, or where the relationship has been short, trust is low. The need for policy specificity varies inversely with trust and experience.

- *Importance:* Significant issues likely to have a large impact on the organization demand greater policy specificity than do issues of lesser probable impact.

- *Risk:* Some activities are inherently more dangerous than others, and the board needs to consider the untoward consequences that could arise if the policy is misinterpreted or inappropriately applied and implemented. The need for specificity varies directly with the degree of risk.

- *Potential of misinterpretation:* Where a directive or limitation could be misinterpreted, greater specificity is warranted.

Everything else being equal (and it never is), boards need to be more specific about their expectations and directives if trust and experience are low, the issue is important, risks are high, and the chance of misinterpretation is great. In such instances, the interpretive and implementive degrees of freedom should be narrowed by constructing a smaller policy box.

Guidelines

Here are some key guidelines for formulating policy:

As policies are a board's most important pronouncements, they must be crafted with great care. Because of their influence, boards have an obligation to be cautious and thoughtful when conveying what they want and expect. A policy is formulated with a hoped-for result in mind; be very clear about what it is. Equally important, consider potential negative and unintended consequences. How could the policy be misinterpreted? What could go wrong?

The best policies are authoritative. They should be expressed powerfully. Equivocal language—words such as "may," "might," "should," and "could"—*must* be avoided. Precision is needed for the board's directives and limitations to be attended to, understood, and heeded.

Policies must be written. They need to be laid out for all to see. Absent written policies, board directives are nothing more than hot air. Additionally, reducing expectations and directives to writing forces precision and clarity.

Policies should be brief. Wordiness confuses rather than clarifies. To be understood and have the desired impact, policies must be easily digested—typically expressed in less than one page.

Policymaking should be minimalistic and parsimonious. This is an arena where less is generally better. Boards should formulate as few policies as necessary to convey what they want and expect in each area of responsibility. The noise caused by too many policies can obscure what is really important.

Policies should be comprehensive. Despite the need for brevity, a board must look at each of its responsibilities and formulate a set of policies that cover the issues, leaving no big gaps. For example, it's ineffective to formulate policies regarding financial objectives without specifying what indicators of financial performance the board will employ to monitor and assess such performance.

Policies must be systematically codified. Exhibit 5.3 provides a form we have found useful for stating policies in a consistent format.

Policies must be compiled and distributed. All of a board's policies must be brought together in one place. We suggest a three-ring binder with five subdivisions—one for each of the board's areas of

```
┌─────────────────────────────────────────────────────────────────────┐
│                                                                       │
│  Responsibility area:              Policy number: _10.2_             │
│  ☐ ends                                                               │
│  ☐ management                      Page _1_ of _1_                    │
│  ☐ quality                                                            │
│  ☐ finances                        Date of origination: _10-25-99_    │
│  ☑ self                                                               │
│                                    Review: _every other year_        │
│  Issue:  _board member conflicts of interest_                         │
│                                                                       │
│  Policy:                                                              │
│  _____ │
│  _____ │
│  _____ │
│  _____ │
│  _____ │
│  _____ │
│  _____ │
│  _____ │
│  _____ │
│  _____ │
│  _____ │
│  _____ │
│  _____ │
│  _____ │
│  _____ │
│                                                                       │
└─────────────────────────────────────────────────────────────────────┘
```

Exhibit 5.3. Policy Codification Form

responsibility. This policy book should then be distributed to each board member, member of the top management team, and medical staff officer. All these copies of the policy book must be kept up to date.

All board policies should be periodically reviewed. Outmoded and outdated policies must be tossed out or modified. We recommend conducting an audit of all board policies at least every other year.

Decision Making

Ask a board member what the most important thing that the board does and the answer you typically get is "make decisions." Decisions, like those illustrated in the sidebar, are important and boards do have to make them. However, board decisions must be grounded on and shaped by policy. That is, a board must first formulate policy in an area of responsibility with respect to a particular issue, and only then consider what needs to be decided. Without this framework, individual decisions run the risk of being idiosyncratic, disjointed, conflicting, and ineffective.

Illustration: Decisions, Decisions

- Should the amount of funds allocated to providing free care be increased next year and, if so, by what amount? (This decision deals with the board's responsibilities for *ends* and *finances*.)

- To what extent did the CEO exceed board specified performance objectives last year? How much of a bonus should be awarded? (This decision deals with the board's responsibility for *executive management performance*.)

- Should Dr. Soandso be reappointed to the medical staff? Should this doctor's privileges be expanded as recommended by the medical staff credentials committee? (This decision deals with the board's responsibility for *quality.*)

- Should the net inpatient operating profit margin objective be increased to 4.5 percent for the next fiscal year? (This decision deals with the board's responsibility for *finances*.)

- Should the size of the board be reduced from twenty-seven to twelve members as recommended by a recently concluded governance assessment? (This decision deals with the board's responsibility for *itself*—its own effectiveness and efficiency.)

Statement	No	Somewhat	Yes
• My board has a formal system in place for formulating and codifying policy.	1	2	3
• My board spends a significant amount of time and energy formulating, deliberating, and debating policy.	1	2	3
• Through the formulation of policies, my board conveys its most important expectations and directives regarding organizational ends.	1	2	3
• Through the formulation of policies, my board conveys its most important expectations and directives regarding executive management performance.	1	2	3
• Through the formulation of policies, my board conveys its most important expectations and directives regarding the quality of care provided in and by the organization.	1	2	3
• Through the formulation of policies, my board conveys its most important expectations and directives regarding the organization's finances.	1	2	3

(continued on page 95)

Statement	No	Somewhat	Yes
• Through the formulation of policies, my board conveys its most important expectations and directives regarding governance contributions and performance.	1	2	3
• At least every other year, we conduct an audit of all board policies to ensure their continued relevance.	1	2	3
TOTAL =			

Governance Check-Up: Policy Formulation
Source: © Dennis D. Pointer, 1998. Adapted from the Governance Assessment Process (GAP)®. Duplication or use beyond the scope of this book is prohibited.

```
8      10      12      14      16      18      20      22      24
```

| Low Performance | Moderate Performance | High Performance |

Board Decision-Making Options

As depicted in Exhibit 5.4, the board has four options for making decisions regarding issues in each of its areas of responsibility.

Option #1: Retaining authority and making the decision itself. For example, boards always retain decisions dealing with their responsibility for themselves—their own structure, composition, and infrastructure.

Option #2: Requesting proposals and recommendations from management or medical staff prior to making a decision. For example, boards make credentialing decisions based on recommendations forwarded by the medical staff.

Option #3: Delegating decision-making authority with constraints. Decisions are handed off to management or the medical staff, but with imposed limitations. For example, the board

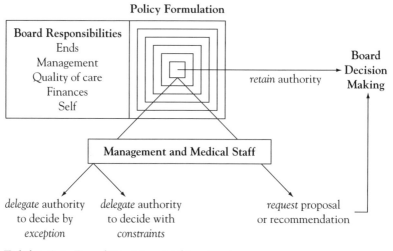

Exhibit 5.4. Board Decision-Making Options

authorizes the CEO to move funds from one budget category to another as long as they are less than a specified amount; if the transfer exceeds this limit, the CEO must seek board approval.

Option #4: Delegating decision making by exception. Management and the medical staff are authorized to make any and all decisions, with the exception of those that have been either expressly prohibited or reserved by the board. In the absence of this option, day-to-day decision making in the organization would come to a complete standstill.

Guidelines

Here are a few key principles that can enhance a board's execution of its decision-making role.

A board should attempt to make as few decisions as possible. This somewhat counterintuitive principle is consistent with the notion that board work should focus on policy, not decision making. As a board pays more attention to policymaking and formulates better policies, the number of decisions it will need to make decreases dra-matically. Policy provides the best mechanism for a board to influ-ence decisions without actually having to make them.

Do not fall into the trap of ratifying decisions that are appropriately within the domain of management and the medical staff. One of the things we see boards doing all the time is redeciding what has already been decided by others. There are two problems here. First, the practice wastes a lot of precious time. Second, when a board rat-ifies a decision that has already (and appropriately) been made by management or the medical staff, it becomes a board decision. Except where required by law or mandated by accreditation crite-ria, this is never warranted.

All proposals should be subject to committee review before being placed on the board's agenda for action. Proposals arrive at the board-room door as complex and weighty documents with important implications for the organization—and if they do not, they should not be placed before the board at all. The reality, in even the very best boards, is that individual members may not have the knowl-edge, expertise, experience, or for that matter patience to evaluate all proposals thoroughly. Consequently, the board's committees must assist the board in its evaluations by investigating, seeking justifi-cation, questioning assumptions, and exploring options prior to board discussion and debate, deliberation, and action.

Only the most important and potentially risky decisions should be retained by the board. It's essential to keep those decisions that can-not be delegated because of legal mandates or functional necessity, as well as those decisions dealing with the most significant aspects of organizational ends and means. The board should request pro-posals prior to making decisions in areas where it does not have the capacity and competence to be proactive. Everything else should be delegated—in the vast majority of instances by exception, and only where absolutely necessary, with imposed constraints.

At the end of the year, a representative sampling of board decisions should be reviewed. Some questions that might be asked: Are

Statement	No	Somewhat	Yes
• My board makes decisions in a timely manner.	1	2	3
• My board has a formal mechanism in place for reviewing and analyzing recommendations and proposals forwarded by management and the medical staff.	1	2	3
• My board does not ratify or approve decisions and actions that are appropriately made by management and the medical staff.	3	2	1
• My board's decision making is policy driven.	1	2	3
• In making decisions, my board often becomes involved in operational matters.	3	2	1
• My board makes too many decisions.	3	2	1
• My board has a way of codifying and disseminating the decisions it makes.	1	2	3
• Each year my board conducts an audit of the appropriateness of decisions it makes.	1	2	3
TOTAL =			

Governance Check-Up: Decision Making

Source: © Dennis D. Pointer, 1998. Adapted from the Governance Assessment Process (GAP)®. Duplication or use beyond the scope of this book is prohibited.

8	10	12	14	16	18	20	22	24

Low Performance	Moderate Performance	High Performance

decisions policy-based and consistent? Are these the type of decisions the board should be making? Did the board have to make these decisions, or could any of them have been better (or more appropriately) made by management or the medical staff? If the board decision dealt with a proposal or recommendation forwarded to it, was a thorough analysis undertaken in committee prior to full board action? Are there types of decisions the board made that could have been avoided if a policy had been in place?

Oversight

The dashboard of your car does not provide a lot of information, but imagine trying to drive without it—no gas gauge, no odometer, no battery or oil pressure indicator lights. Feedback is essential for altering what you do and how you do it, both immediately and over the long run. Nonetheless, most boards attempt to govern their organizations without well-designed dashboards containing the right gauges. Driving partially blind, they do not have the information they need to tell whether things are working out as expected and planned.

Nature of the Role

In executing its oversight role, a board monitors and assesses key organizational processes and outcomes. This accountability assurance mechanism provides the means to answer four questions: Is the organization performing in a manner that protects and advances stakeholder interests? Are board expectations, as conveyed in its policies, being met? Are board decisions having the desired impact? Are the board's directives and constraints being respected as management and the medical staff perform delegated tasks?

As illustrated in Exhibit 5.5, there are five aspects of the oversight process.

Selecting indicators: There are any number of things a board can choose to monitor and assess. What should it focus its

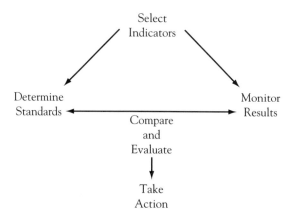

Exhibit 5.5. The Oversight Process

attention upon? What must a board oversee to ensure accountability and get the feedback it needs to govern effectively?

Specifying standards: With respect to each indicator, what does the board expect? What constitutes exemplary, adequate, or unacceptable levels of performance?

Monitoring results: For each indicator, it is necessary to gather data that answers the question, What actually happened?

Comparing results with standards: How does performance stack up against established standards?

Taking action: What should be done if there is a difference between results and expectations?

Illustration: Board Oversight

- *Indicator:* nonexempt employee turnover

  Standard: less than 15 percent of adjusted FTEs per year

  Monitored result: 12.2 percent for the most recent year end

Comparison: standard exceeded

Action: celebrate and reward

- *Indicator:* Inpatient operating profit margin

  Standard: 5 percent of adjusted gross revenues

  Monitored result: 3.5 percent

  Comparison: a difference of −1.5 percent; standard
  was not met

  Action: request plan from management to correct
  the problem

- *Indicator:* average regularly scheduled board meeting
  absentee rate

  Standard: not to exceed 12 percent

  Monitored result: 22 percent

  Comparison: standard not met

  Action: attendance record to be distributed to all board members quarterly; chairperson to meet with members who have
  missed more than four meetings in the last year and discuss
  their participation

Governance Information

Most boards do not suffer from a lack of information—they are
inundated, often overwhelmed, by it. Unfortunately, the wrong type
of information is often presented in the wrong way. Boards typically
receive products of the organization's management and clinical
information systems. These systems have been designed to support
management and medical staff work. Boards have different responsibilities and roles from those of executives and physicians; to do
their work they need governance, not operational, information. The
design of governance information systems, an important aspect of
a board's infrastructure, is addressed in Chapter Eight. We focus here
on the products of such systems and how they should facilitate
board oversight.

Boards must take the initiative in specifying the type of information they need to execute their oversight role. Although management and the medical staff must be involved, this responsibility rests squarely with the board; only it can specify the information required to oversee the organization in a way that ensures accountability.

Returning to the automobile analogy, what dashboards are needed? In executing its oversight role, how should the board's very limited attention, time, and energy be focused? We recommend five dashboards—one for each responsibility. Boards are responsible for ensuring organizational ends, high levels of executive management performance, quality of care, financial health, and their own effectiveness and efficiency. Overseeing the extent to which these responsibilities have been fulfilled closes the loop with respect to the what and how of governance.

For each dashboard, an appropriate number and type of gauges (indicators) must be constructed. What specific aspects of the organization's performance should be monitored? We suggest that the answer, although idiosyncratic, is determined by a board's responsibilities and the policies that convey expectations regarding them. At minimum, a set of indicators and gauges must be developed for the following:

Ends	The extent to which the vision is being fulfilled and key goals are being accomplished
Management	The extent to which the CEO's performance is in line with board expectations
Finances	The extent to which the organization's financial performance is in line with board-specified objectives and expectations
Quality	The extent to which quality of care (as defined by the board) meets standards
Self	The extent to which the board is fulfilling its responsibilities and executing its roles

The selection of indicator gauges is based on a board's key expectations. The principle:

If something is important enough for a board to express an expectation about, it is important enough to monitor.

Guidelines

If a board expectation is so trivial and unimportant that it does not need to be tracked and assessed, it should not have been expressed in the first place. When a board attempts to monitor too many things, it will monitor nothing well. Accordingly, we recommend that fewer than twenty indicator gauges be developed for each responsibility.

A standard must be attached to each indicator, specifying what a board wants. If the basic principle is followed (a board's most important expectations drive the selection of indicators), then the matter of standard specification is easily solved—an expectation typically contains within it a standard. For example, consider a typical board policy regarding financial performance: "Net operating margin from inpatient operations should exceed 5 percent." The indicator is net inpatient operating margin. The standard is 5 percent.

The indicators must be quantitative, or quantifiable. If something is not measurable, it cannot be monitored. It is important to note that most subjective measures of performance can be quantified. For example, the level of physician satisfaction with the quality of nursing care can be quantified through an appropriately designed, administered, and analyzed questionnaire.

Monitored results for each indicator must be comparative. By far the most meaningful and useful information has a high degree of contrast. When data on indicators is presented across time, juxtaposed against a standard, or compared with like institutions, trends and patterns are more easily identified and interpreted.

Remember that data only becomes information when it is organized. And the best method of organization is a graph. The old adage is true: a picture is worth a thousand words (or columns of data).

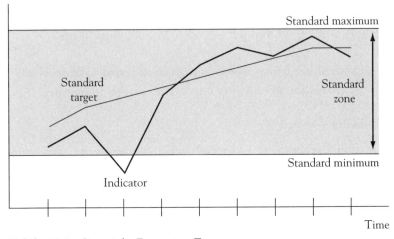

Exhibit 5.6. Oversight Reporting Format
Source: Adapted from Pointer and Ewell, 1994.

Picture the product of a board's governance information system as a three-ring binder. There are five dividers labeled Ends, Management, Quality, Finances, and Self. Behind each divider there are less than twenty pieces of paper, each reflecting a separate indicator that has been selected by the board to measure performance with respect to its most important expectations. The pages in each section follow a common format, as illustrated in Exhibit 5.6.

An indicator that captures a key board expectation is portrayed across some period of time and contrasted against a standard (which could be a target, ceiling, floor, or zone). The board, with assistance of its standing committees in each area, reviews the indicators and associated standards quarterly. If the standard is not met, the board requests management or medical staff to devise a plan to address and correct the problem.

Benchmark Practices: Roles

- We find that most boards spend upwards of 50 percent of their meeting time listening to reports—from management, from the medical staff, from board committees. The habit of devoting large

Statement	No	Somewhat	Yes
• My board has developed a set of quantitative indicators and standards to monitor and assess how well our organization is accomplishing key goals and fulfilling its vision.	1	2	3
• My board has developed a set of quantitative indicators and standards to monitor and assess executive management performance.	1	2	3
• My board has developed a set of quantitative indicators and standards to monitor and assess the quality of care provided in and by our organization.	1	2	3
• My board has developed a set of quantitative indicators and standards to monitor and assess the organization's financial health.	1	2	3
• We have developed a set of quantitative indicators and standards to monitor and assess the board's own performance and contributions.	1	2	3
• At least quarterly, my board monitors and assesses key indicators and standards in each of its areas of responsibility.	1	2	3

(continued on page 106)

Governance Check-Up: Oversight

Statement	No	Somewhat	Yes
• When such review and assessment indicates there are problems, a mechanism is in place to ensure that management or medical staff will correct them.	1	2	3
• My board periodically assesses the standards and indicators it employs to ensure their continued relevance.	1	2	3
TOTAL =			

Governance Check-Up: Oversight
Source: © Dennis D. Pointer, 1998. Adapted from the Governance Assessment Process (GAP)®. Duplication or use beyond the scope of this book is prohibited.

8	10	12	14	16	18	20	22	24

Low
Performance

Moderate
Performance

High
Performance

amounts of time to passive listening is one of the biggest barriers boards face in transforming how they govern in ways that significantly enhance their performance and contributions. Clearly, some listening is necessary. But much of what boards listen to is marginally important, redundant, or could be conveyed in other (and much more efficient) ways. Board meeting time is very limited. The best boards use most of this precious time for deliberating and debating and formulating policy, considering and making decisions, and overseeing organizational performance and outcomes. These boards create and jealously protect the amount of time needed to execute their governance roles by severely restricting the time they spend just listening.

•   Passive listening is not the only problem for a board. Exhibit 5.7 denotes how the typical board allocates whatever attention, time, and effort it has available, over and above the time spent listening to things it doesn't need to hear. (Not all listening time is wasted time, of course, but it does all need to be questioned to see if it's worthwhile.) The exhibit also illustrates how a board employing best practices allocates its much greater amount of available time.

The typical board spends the vast majority of its nonlistening time making decisions, about 20 percent engaged in oversight, and 10 percent formulating policy. The best boards have a very different profile: They spend more than half of their time deliberating, debating, and formulating policy, about 30 percent engaged in oversight, and less than 20 percent making decisions. That is, the best boards recognize what we have been preaching throughout this chapter—governance must be policy driven. A board's most important role is to convey expectations on behalf of stakeholders, ensuring their interests and needs are protected and advanced by the organization. The most effective and efficient way for a board to do this is to avoid immersing itself in mountains of organizational

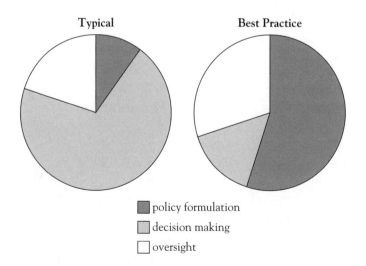

Exhibit 5.7. How Boards Spend Their Time

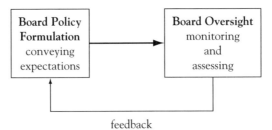

Exhibit 5.8. Benchmark Governance

detail, and instead to craft the context in which management and the medical staff act and decide by formulating policies and then overseeing the results. We do not want to deprecate decision making—it is a necessary aspect of board work, but the center of gravity of benchmark governance can be simply diagramed (see Exhibit 5.8).

By formulating policy a board conveys its most important expectations (regarding ends, executive management performance, quality, finances, and its own behavior) on behalf of the organization's stakeholders. The board then monitors performance and outcomes to ensure that these expectations are being fulfilled (by itself, by management, by the medical staff). Oversight provides the feedback employed by a board to adjust (and fine-tune) its expectations and the way they are conveyed.

Benchmark Practices: Policy Formulation

• Realize that your board does not need (and should not want) to formulate all its policies overnight. Starting from scratch, it takes most boards a year or more to craft and convey their most important expectations and directives. This is an area that rewards quality of the activity, not speed.

• Settle on a form that your board will employ to codify its policies (the one in Exhibit 5.3 can be adapted to any environment).

• Remember the "perils of perfection." Attempting to formulate perfect policies will sabotage your effort.

- Scan your present board polices (whether separately codified or embedded in board meeting minutes) and policy-related documents; eliminate those that are not truly important or necessary. Use this scan to identify policies (or policy-like statements) that warrant being rewritten or formally codified, and then do so.

- Start by formulating the easiest policies first. In most cases, these are ones dealing with the board's responsibility regarding its own performance and contributions. What are your board's most important expectations of itself? Consider such areas as conflicts of interest, confidentiality, board member education and development, and meeting attendance. You might want to draft a board job description or charter using the illustrative sidebar provided in this chapter as a point of departure.

- Once you have some policies regarding the board's own work, start working on those dealing with management performance and finances. Again, do not attempt to write all policies in each of these areas—focus on only the very most important board expectations and directives, those most critical "thou shalts" and "shalt nots." Begin by specifying key CEO performance expectations and financial objectives.

- Leave the formulation of policies dealing with ends until much later in the process. Conventional wisdom suggests that they should be developed first as all other policies are supposed to be grounded on, and flow from, the board's vision and key goals. True, but policies regarding an organization's ends are by far the toughest and most time-consuming to formulate; starting with them is generally frustrating and can derail your board's effort to become policy driven. You can always revisit your first attempts at policymaking and refine them as needed after you codify your ends.

- Use committees to assist your board in formulating policies. We suggest the following steps:

1. A committee (for example, the finance committee for policies dealing with finances) develops a list of the most important things that policies need to be formulated about.

2. Time is scheduled at a board meeting to discuss one of the areas on the list, outline the general parameters of a policy, and sketch the board's key expectations and directives.

3. The committee then prepares a draft policy based on the board's discussion.

4. The committee's draft policy is placed on the board's agenda for deliberation and debate, modification, and vote. The process continues until each of the areas on all of the committee's lists have been considered.

Benchmark Practices: Oversight

• The process for developing oversight mechanisms should be fundamentally different from the one employed for formulating policy. We recommend that your board construct a full (though less than fully polished and refined) dashboard of indicators. That is, go for breadth first, and then continually embellish, elaborate, and refine over time.

• Consider appointing a board task force (which should include members of management and the medical staff and a few outsiders as well). The committee's charge is to identify key indicators on which data is already being collected in the organization (through the managerial and clinical information systems) that could be employed by your board to oversee the extent to which ends are being achieved, the performance of executive management, the quality of care, the organization's financial health, and the board's own performance and contributions. We recommend initially identifying no more than a dozen potential indicators in each area or responsibility.

• Hold a mini-retreat, special board meeting, or working session dedicated exclusively to oversight design. During this session, the board can review the committee's lists of indicators and construct an initial governance dashboard. We suggest that no more that five or six gauges be included for each responsibility.

• Over the following six months, your board should practice "fly-ing by instruments"—using the dashboard to perform its oversight role. Here are the key aspects of the process:

> *Step 1:* Committees review indicators within their scope of responsibility.
>
> *Step 2:* Full board reviews and discusses key indicators for each core responsibility.
>
> *Step 3:* When Step 2 surfaces indicators that reveal areas when the organization is not meeting standards, the board requests corrective plans from management or medical staff.
>
> *Step 4:* Committees and the full board follow up as necessary.

• Once your board has some experience with the process, we sug-gest that you circle back and begin to refine and expand the indi-cators for each responsibility area. This task should be delegated to the appropriate committees (for example, the board's finance com-mittee tackles financial indicators, the quality committee focuses on quality of care indicators, and so on). Keep in mind that the task is not to identify every possible indicator, just the most critical ones that the board must monitor and assess. Indicators should be linked to the board's most important expectations—its policies. The process is an ongoing one—indicators should be added or deleted as circumstances and challenges change.

Essence of the Phrase *To Govern*

This and the previous chapter have focused on board functioning, the responsibilities to which boards must attend and the roles they must perform. How a board chooses to function—the way it allo-cates its precious and very limited attention, time, and energy—more than any other factor, will determine its performance and contributions.

To make a difference and add value on behalf of stakeholders, a board must have a shared, coherent, and empowering answer to the fundamental question of governance: *What type of work should we be doing?* Our answer to this question is portrayed in Exhibit 5.9.

Boards must formulate policy, make decisions, and engage in oversight with respect to ends, executive management performance, quality of care, finances, and their own practices; this is the essence of the phrase "to govern."

We recommend boards put into writing their own definition of what it means to govern. The sidebar gives an example.

Illustration: Board Charter

It is our board's obligation to ensure the organization's resources are deployed in a manner that protects and advances stakeholder interests. To fulfill this obligation, we formulate policy (convey expectations, direct, and guide), make decisions (choose among alternatives) and oversee (monitor and assess) ends, executive management performance, quality of care, finances, and our board's own performance and contributions.

Our board is responsible for determining the organization's ends. To fulfill this responsibility, we formulate the organization's vision, its core values, and its purposes. We also specify key goals designed to lead to fulfillment of the vision, and review strategies devised by management to make sure that they are aligned with key goals and the vision.

Our board is responsible for ensuring high levels of executive management performance. To fulfill this responsibility, we select and recruit the chief executive officer (CEO); formulate CEO performance objectives; appraise the CEO's performance; determine the CEO's compensation; and, should the need arise, terminate the CEO's relationship with the organization. Subject to its directives and oversight, the board delegates all management functions to the CEO. The CEO

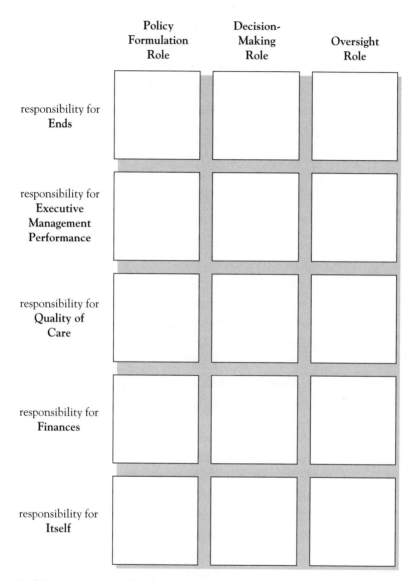

Exhibit 5.9. Board Work

Source: Adapted from Pointer and Ewell, 1994.

is the only employee directly accountable to the board for management of the organization.

Our board is responsible for ensuring the quality of care provided in and by the organization. To fulfill this responsibility, we define what quality health care means; appoint, reappoint, and determine privileges of medical staff members; ensure necessary quality and utilization monitoring systems are in place and functioning effectively; and determine quality standards and employ them to assess the care provided.

Our board is responsible for the organization's financial health, and protecting and enhancing the community's investment in it. To fulfill this responsibility, we establish financial objectives, ensure financial planning is undertaken in a manner that leads to accomplishing such objectives, monitor and assess financial performance, and ensure necessary control mechanisms are in place.

We are responsible for our own effectiveness and efficiency. To fulfill this responsibility, our board ensures that it is discharging its responsibilities and roles, its structure is appropriate, its members possess the knowledge and skills needed to govern, and the necessary systems and procedures are in place to assist them in doing their work.

6

Governance Structure

When we speak at conferences on the topic of governance structure, boredom tends to set in. Eyes glaze over as we discuss the many different structural alternatives and their implications. Yet many of the panicked calls we get from clients deal with these very same issues.

What a board does is clearly more important than *how* it does it. Form, after all, should follow function. However, our consulting experience strongly suggests that inappropriate structure is one of the most common causes of less than optimal governance performance and contributions.

Governance structure involves all aspects of the form of a board or boards, including the size of the board and the number and type of board committees. In health care organizations with multiple boards, structure also deals with the number of boards, their relationships, and their relative responsibilities and roles.

Although the ideal governance structure for health care organizations is hotly debated, one thing is clear: many boards are attempting to confront twenty-first-century challenges with governance structures designed for earlier and more forgiving times.

Some health care organizations have too many boards. (While it is theoretically possible to have too few boards, we have rarely seen this as a problem.) Some boards have too many members, while some boards have too few. Often, boards have too many committees. In an all too common role reversal, many boards are controlled by their committees. Some boards have no control over the selection of their members, others are required to use representational selection processes.

Whatever form it takes, inefficient governance structure inhibits effective governance functioning, often resulting in gridlock. A cumbersome, slow decision-making process (often due to the multiplicity of boards or committees) causes confusion in authority, responsibilities, and roles. Consensus-based decision making is often the default setting, which results in a slow governance process that is unable to deal effectively with markets undergoing revolutionary change. In addition to gridlock, governance conflict occurs when different boards or committees within an organization actually fight over who has the authority to make decisions or to address specific issues. We have seen different boards within a system attempt to assert their authority by making intentionally incompatible decisions. This is hardly governance at its best.

Ineffective governance structure always squanders the most precious of all leadership resources: time. Excessive and inappropriate consumption of board time can cause member burnout. Further, excessive and irrelevant consumption of executive management time by governance robs the organization of critical guidance and operational control by deflecting management attention to marginal issues. Opportunities slip away, delays in decision making paralyze the organization, and frustration increases exponentially.

But this issue is not simply important in terms of avoiding the negative consequences of inefficient structures. While it is true that ineffective governance structure generally leads to ineffective functioning, the reverse is also true: efficient governance structure promotes effective functioning. The right structure is necessary to provide a liberating framework for the creativity, imagination, focus, big-picture thinking, and timely and meaningful action that is the hallmark of good governance.

Issues in System Governance Structure

Any discussion of governance structure must first address the issue of the structure of multiple-governance entities: those health care organizations that have more than one board, a common characteristic of multihospital and integrated delivery systems. These multiple boards exist within the same organization and have superior-subordinate relationships. Fully 65 percent of hospital boards report that they are responsible to a higher authority (American Hospital Association, 1997).

Perspective: Layers of Governance

Governance structure has a *breadth* dimension and a *depth* dimension. Governance breadth is the number of boards in a health care organization. Depth refers to the number of layers of governance—the hierarchy of governance reporting relationships.

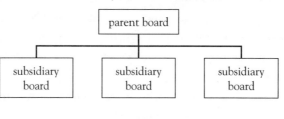

Two Layers of Governance

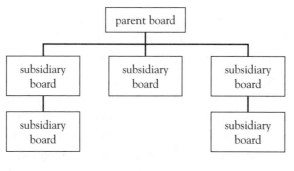

Three Layers of Governance

Multiple governance organizations are the rule rather than the exception in the health care industry. Even a stand-alone hospital often has more than one board: a parent board, a hospital board, a foundation board, and related boards such as a physician-hospital organization board are all quite commonly found together. All integrated delivery systems with which we have worked and are familiar have had multiple boards, although some have since abandoned them. For these organizations to function effectively, it is absolutely critical that the relative responsibilities and roles of each governance entity be clearly defined and well understood. It is equally important that the structure of these multiple layers of boards be thoughtfully designed to facilitate effective governance.

One Board or Many?

Health care systems, whether called integrated delivery systems, organized delivery systems, or some other name, can be defined in a number of ways—but one fundamental characteristic is that they are composed of two or more organizations. These can include hospitals, nursing homes, insurance companies, physician groups, outpatient surgery centers, rehabilitation facilities, and home care agencies—and the list could go on to cover the whole health care field.

As systems have added subsidiary organizations, many have simultaneously added additional boards or board committees to help govern them. The governance structures of many of these systems have become bloated and cumbersome, adding costs that far exceed their value. A number of systems have initiated restructuring projects to streamline their governance and improve their functioning. We have participated in many of these projects over the years, and our ideas and perspectives are drawn from such experiences.

There are three basic models of system governance structure: centralized, decentralized, and modified centralized. Exhibits 6.1 and 6.2 illustrate the first two; the third is a combination of the others with too many variations to encompass in one drawing.

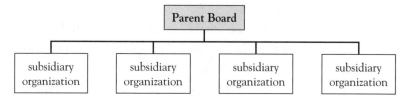

Exhibit 6.1. Centralized Governance Structure

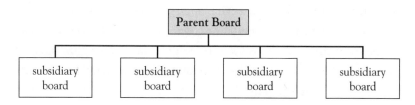

Exhibit 6.2. Decentralized Governance Structure

In a *centralized structure* the organization is governed by a single board exercising ultimate authority over all subsidiaries directly. Subsidiary organizations are not governed by separate boards, although they may have advisory bodies that exercise no legal or fiduciary authority.

The *decentralized governance structure* is defined by multiple boards and layers of governance. The parent board retains authority and reserved powers over subsidiary boards, but governance responsibilities and roles are subdivided and shared. One of the responsibilities of the parent is oversight and coordination of subsidiary boards. In the decentralized governance structure, delineation and sharing of authority and functions among the different boards is an issue of critical importance.

The third model is a hybrid of the first two. A *modified centralized structure* has a parent board and as few subsidiary boards as possible (usually three or fewer). This model is technically no different from the second in that there is more than one board. But it is functionally different in that it is a streamlined structure, with a deliberate attempt to limit the number of boards and carefully artic-ulate and coordinate their functioning. The vast majority of health care organizations currently employ some type of multiple-board governance structure, either decentralized or modified centralized.

We are, however, familiar with a very few health care organiza-tions that have adopted a single-board, centralized approach to gov-ernance. The potential benefits of such a model include the facilitation of rapid and effective decision making and the reduc-tion of executive time devoted to governance. Additionally, a sin-gle board is more likely to focus on appropriate big-picture issues, as it would be very difficult for it to meddle in the details of a mod-erate to fairly large system.

A single-board, centralized governance structure presents cer-tain difficulties as well. These include a limitation on the number of community members and other stakeholders that can participate in governance as compared to a multiple-board organization. Fur-ther, having a single board govern a complex, far-flung system car-ries some risk that the board may become too far removed from effective oversight and rely excessively on management, which could result in management domination or manipulation of the board. Another risk is that the board's time may be consumed by required, detail-oriented functions such as approving medical staff credentials and receiving and approving reports that are mandated by legislation and regulators.

The decentralized model allows a parent board to assign certain responsibilities to subsidiary boards. The subsidiary boards can then focus on their communities and organizations, presumably allow-ing the parent board to focus on systemwide issues. As a decentral-ized model also results in many boards, it creates many board seats to be filled. This provides the opportunity to involve a larger num-ber of community members, physicians, and other stakeholders in governance.

While decentralized governance is by far the most common model, we believe that its many and significant disadvantages far outweigh its potential benefits. This model often results in dysfunctional governance primarily because of the overly cumbersome decision-making process it creates. Responsibilities and roles of multiple boards are often unclear, which can often result in tension or conflict between them. Multiple boards often consume inordinate amounts of executive management's time and energy.

Perhaps the greatest argument against the decentralized model, however, is its tendency to generate representational governance. If subsidiary boards represent the interests of "their" organizations, as opposed to the interests of the system as a whole, the whole system suffers—including the subsidiary organizations.

The third model, the modified centralized governance structure, has the potential to provide many of the advantages of both the centralized and decentralized approaches. This model, through a few carefully chosen subsidiary boards, can allow the parent to focus on systemwide issues while referring oversight of specific regions, organizations, or lines of business to other groups that have the time and attention span to do justice to the issues involved.

Just as the modified centralized model can provide a combination of the benefits of the first two models, it also has the obvious potential to result in the worst of them as well. Representational governance, gridlock, limited board seats for community and stakeholder involvement, as well as excessive consumption of management time are all possible negative consequences of this model.

Each model, centralized, decentralized, and modified centralized has its own strengths and weaknesses, but our bias is streamlined governance. However, the most common structural model, by far, is the decentralized. We like this model the least of the three; in practice, its disadvantages always outweigh its benefits. The vast majority of our governance restructuring consulting projects result in transformation of an existing decentralized model of governance into a modified centralized model—or occasionally even a pure centralized one.

We recommend a modified centralized or, if possible, a pure centralized model of governance.

Subsidiary Board Structure

Our recommendations notwithstanding, we recognize that the most common governance model for systems is the decentralized one. Structural issues are far from resolved when one model is chosen. In either the decentralized or the modified centralized model, governance responsibilities and roles must still be divided among the multiple subsidiary boards. There are three basic ways this can be done—organizational, regional, and functional—although some combination of the three is also often feasible.

In an *organizational* model (Exhibit 6.3), every organization in a system is governed by a separate subsidiary board. Thus, if a system had five hospitals, a nursing home, an insurance company, a visiting nurses agency (VNA), and a medical group, the system would have a total of ten boards: one system board, five hospital boards, one nursing home board, one insurance company board, one VNA board, and one medical group board.

A decentralized governance model with subsidiary boards for each organization is by far the most common model of system governance. It is the default setting for most systems, evolving on its own simply because little thought has been given to governance structure in the nascent stages of system formation. Even though this model is the most common one, we believe it is also the worst.

The decentralized model promotes representational governance. Frequently, the parent board will be composed of representatives from the subsidiary boards. This can create a belief that the primary purpose of subsidiary board members on the parent board is to represent the interests of their sponsoring subsidiary, and only secondarily—if at all—to represent the best interests of the system as a whole. This representative emphasis inhibits the ability of the par-

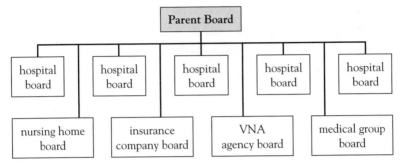

Exhibit 6.3. The Organizational Model

ent board to govern the entire system effectively, and to control and coordinate subsidiary boards.

Perspective: The Trap of Decentralized Governance

A medical group and a small hospital join forces, keeping their own boards in addition to placing people on a central board mandated to look after their combined operations. After all, they both want to gain by the association—not lose anything, including the specialized expertise they each bring to their own operations. They work well together, and the structure feels both logical and manageable. Then they pick up a medical laboratory, then another hospital joins them. They all prosper together, and other organizations attach themselves to the growing power—all following the practice of the original partners and retaining their own boards while adding members to the central board. After a while, the central board finds that it is too busy listening to reports, mediating among the boards of the member organizations, and debating trivia to attend to the organization's place and role in the community it serves. Further, the system CEO spends an inordinate amount of time attending many different board meetings.

We have seen some small to medium-sized systems with over thirty boards! In each of these cases the CEO and system board chair were at a loss to explain how this top-heavy governance arrangement had occurred. "We just grew into it" or "It just happened" are common explanations. This model universally demands inordinate amounts of management time and risks conflict between subsidiary boards.

Perhaps the greatest drawback of this model is that as the system grows, so does the number of subsidiary boards; each organization created or acquired by the system will have its own. Further, if every subsidiary board has a representative on the parent board, as the number of subsidiaries grows, the parent board's size must also grow—soon to a bloated, unmanageable number of members.

In the *regional* model (Exhibit 6.4) of decentralized or modified centralized governance, subsidiary boards are created for each geographic region or market in which the system operates. Each board is responsible for governing all the system's organizations in that particular region.

This model is really only an option for those systems that cover large or sharply divergent geographic regions, and that have strate-

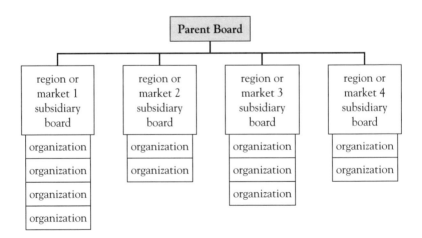

Exhibit 6.4. The Regional or Market Model

gically chosen to divide their activities, organizations, and resources along regional lines. For these systems, this approach has potential in that it can result in a minimal number of boards within a decentralized governance structure. Further, it allows for community and stakeholder representation on regional boards. Finally, if there is a clear and precise division of relative responsibilities and roles between parent and subsidiary boards, this model can allow the parent to focus on systemwide matters while delegating governance issues better handled locally to subsidiary boards.

The regional model, however, has the potential to create significant variation in system operation, quality, and cost efficiency—the antithesis of systemness. It also has the potential to create representational governance on a regional level. We believe the regional model to be a workable one, but with limited applicability to a few very large, geographically dispersed systems. Of the three models, it is our second choice.

Our favorite approach for organizing subsidiary boards in a decentralized or modified centralized governance structure is a *functional* model (Exhibit 6.5). Here, subsidiary boards are created to govern groupings of organizations performing similar functions

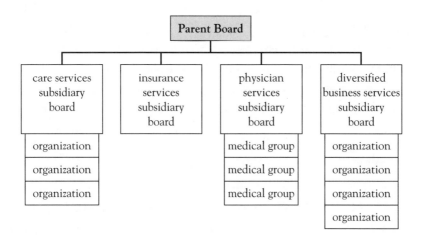

Exhibit 6.5. The Functional Model

(such as institutional care, medical care, insurance, and so on). In this model, the subsidiary boards are not based on what organizations the system has or what regions the system serves, but rather on what the system does.

Just as a health care system can do a variety of things, it can govern on the basis of what it does: care delivery (the entire continuum of care, not just limited to hospital care); physician care; and insurance and managed care services. In a decentralized, functional governance model, a large system might then have four boards, a parent and three subsidiaries; one to govern care delivery functions, one to govern physician groups, and one to govern the insurance company. Or the system might have one subordinate board to oversee all the hospitals within the system and one to oversee all the nursing homes or other delivery organizations.

The functional approach allows a system to adopt a modified centralized governance model with a minimum number of boards. Or it can allow a system with a decentralized model to more logically and coherently organize its subsidiary boards. Under this model there are no artificial distinctions of governance based on buildings, organizations, or regions. Rather, subsidiary boards are organized to govern functions that must be performed.

This model, however, can have many of the same weaknesses of the other two. Representational governance may rear its ugly head. It may inhibit the system from operating smoothly across the continuum of the different functions. Nevertheless, with a bit of effort and coordination, these weaknesses can be minimized. We believe that if a system chooses a decentralized or modified centralized model of governance, the functional approach to governing subsidiary organizations is best.

When we present this recommendation, some executives or board leaders ask whether functional divisions within a system aren't just as artificial as organizational or regional divisions. And they're right—the answer is an unequivocal yes! Functional distinctions are indeed artificial at some level, especially for a mature system that is truly integrated. Systems at that level of maturity may be ready to move to centralized governance, with a single board. This raises an interesting notion. Perhaps the different governance structures represent evolutionary stages that systems pass through as they mature and integrate (see Exhibit 6.6).

The first stage is a decentralized, organization-based structure. The second stage is a modified decentralized model, based either on regions (or markets) or on functions. Here, two variations are possible: the organization implements either a region-market or function-based model, or it moves from a region and market to a functional model. The final stage is centralized governance. Whether this theory is valid or not, many systems pass through stages as they grow and mature. This suggests that different governance structures may be appropriate for systems based on their levels of maturity and integration. It also speaks to the need to recognize that structural models are only appropriate as long as they provide value to a system, and that governance structure must be regularly evaluated and modified as circumstances change.

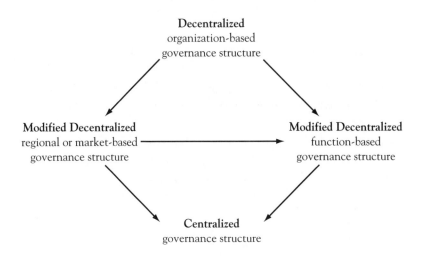

Exhibit 6.6. The Evolution of Governance Structure

Of course, more complex hybrid governance structure models are possible. We have seen systems that actually combine the regional, organizational, and functional approaches to decentralized governance, as illustrated in Exhibit 6.7.

Employing such an approach, the organization has a parent board and some subsidiary regional boards, which in turn have organizational boards subordinate to them. We have also seen this arrangement exist in addition to a functional insurance board subordinate to the parent board and governing an insurance company that provides services in all the regions. Clearly, this represents a very complex governance structure, and one that has the potential to add more cost than value.

To repeat our bias, we favor a centralized model of governance for systems. If this is not practical, we recommend a modified centralized model with subsidiary boards organized along functional lines. We believe that the most common model, the decentralized organizational model, is counterproductive to effective system gov-

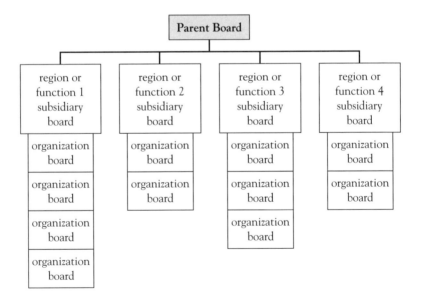

Exhibit 6.7. Hybrid Governance Structures

ernance functioning. We also strongly recommend that governance structure be consistent with management and clinical structures. It does not make sense to have a system with centralized management and clinical operations and decentralized governance.

Our recommendations and biases notwithstanding, we recognize that governance structure, in and of itself, does not create high levels of governance performance and contributions. It either supports or inhibits it. We have seen systems with cumbersome combined governance structures where governance was excellent. Conversely, we have also seen streamlined structures where governance was inadequate. With time, effort, and money any governance structure can be made to work. Nonetheless, not all structures facilitate the most effective governance functioning in the most efficient way.

Other Structural Approaches to Subsidiary Boards

The preceding section presented the most logical ways to structure governance and organize subsidiary boards. These are not the only approaches, however. Here are some of the more common approaches for squeezing centralized governance functioning out of a decentralized structure.

Mirror Boards

As Exhibit 6.8 illustrates, a mirror board is where individuals who make up one board (say a parent) are also the same individuals who make up a subsidiary board. The phrase *mirror board* simply means that the composition of two or more boards is identical. Mirror boards are common in health care organizations.

In certain situations there are legal or regulatory requirements that call for multiple boards. For example, to take advantage of Medicare reimbursement rates, many systems maintain nursing homes as separate corporations, which are required to have their own boards. Further, there are certain state-specific requirements that mandate separate boards for particular types of businesses (common examples are insurance companies and medical groups).

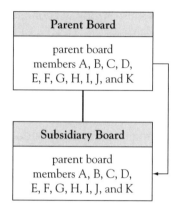

Exhibit 6.8. Mirror Boards

Where there is a legal or regulatory requirement to have multiple boards, but where centralized governance is desired, the use of the mirror board can sometimes address both demands. When a mirror board approach is used, there are legally two boards, but practically only one.

There are drawbacks to mirror boards. To fulfill legal requirements, both boards must hold meetings, keep separate minutes, and take such action as required in their charters and by-laws. The distinction in responsibilities and roles between the two boards can easily become diffuse or confused. Because of this tendency, the mirror approach should never be used with more than two boards. In other words, a parent board and three subsidiary boards, all comprising the same people, may be legal, but it will probably be ineffective.

There may be legal requirements that mandate that the system and subsidiary boards have materially different composition from one another, which precludes the pure mirror board approach. The *adulterated mirror board* approach, illustrated in Exhibit 6.9, responds to this prohibition by placing a few outside members on the subsidiary board. If allowable, a majority of the subsidiary board's mem-

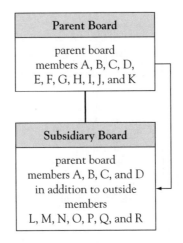

Exhibit 6.9. Adulterated Mirror Board

bers are drawn from the parent. While there are technically two boards with different membership, there are enough members from the parent serving on the subsidiary board to control it.

When a subsidiary board is required to have a majority of members who do not sit on the parent board, another variation on the mirror board approach is possible: the *executive committee mirror,* illustrated in Exhibit 6.10. Here, the executive committees of the parent and subsidiary boards mirror each other. The executive committee mirror approach requires that the executive committee dominate the subsidiary board. A common consequence is a two-class system of governance; members of the subsidiary board who are not on the executive committee come to resent the fact that the real power rests with the executive committee.

We have occasionally found the basic mirror board approach to be necessary and give it a qualified recommendation. In certain situations—where more than one board is required but only one board is desired—this approach, if legally permissible, might be considered. We strongly advise against the executive committee mirror approach, however, as it almost always causes problems.

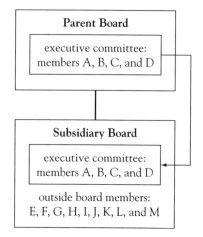

Exhibit 6.10. Executive Committee Mirror Board

Phantom Subordinate Boards

Another way to get centralized governance out of a decentralized structure involves the parent board's limiting the subsidiary board meeting frequency to a fraction of its own. The idea is that if the parent board meets monthly and the subsidiary board meets quarterly (we have even seen some meet annually), the subsidiary board may technically exist but has no practical leverage on the organization. This approach can have value if the subsidiary board's responsibilities and roles are very tightly defined and limited so that it can actually effectively discharge them with infrequent meetings.

Internal Management Boards

Yet another approach to having centralized governance functioning with decentralized structure is the internal management board technique. Here, a subsidiary board is composed of a small number of executives from the parent organization. This board meets infrequently, has very defined and limited responsibilities and roles, and is tightly controlled by the parent board. This approach has a major drawback. If the subsidiary board governs a nonprofit organization, then IRS regulations prohibit executive management or other insiders (such as physicians who do business with the organization) from holding more than 49 percent of the board seats. So the pure internal management board approach cannot be used for a nonprofit subsidiary. However, the internal management subsidiary board can be employed in for-profits. In this situation, the internal management board with reserved power resting with the parent can be quite effective at streamlining a decentralized structure.

Of course, a hybrid approach can be used for a subsidiary board governing a nonprofit. In this approach, a small subsidiary board is composed of 49 percent internal management personnel and 51 percent outsiders. Combining this with the mirror board approach, all or a majority of the 51 percent outsider subsidiary board members can be members of the parent (if legally permissible). Voilà! Two boards but really only one. Add to this a reduced subsidiary board meeting frequency, and we have yet another approach to producing the advantages of centralized governance within a decentralized structure.

Board Size

The number of members of a board is often regarded as the most critical structural governance characteristic. While we don't necessarily agree, board size is nonetheless significant. Large boards (those with more than twenty members) were very useful in the past, when a board's key role was raising funds for the organization it theoretically governed. Well into the 1970s, it was not uncommon to find philanthropic boards of health care organizations with as many as seventy-five members!

Today, except for foundations, philanthropy is not the primary role of health care organization governance, and so having a large board for this express purpose is not necessary. Other common reasons for having a large board include providing an opportunity for significant community involvement in governance, providing for constituency or sponsor participation in governance, and being able to spread an overly burdensome amount of board work (a symptom of ineffective governance in itself) among many members.

Boards with more than twenty members have several structural strikes against them. First, larger boards are more cumbersome decision-making bodies than smaller ones. Second, in an attempt to combat this, large boards tend to have active executive committees that function as the real board by meeting often and discharging most governance responsibilities and roles. This creates a two-class governance system, discussed earlier, with all its attendant problems. Third, larger boards tend to reduce the involvement and consequently diffuse the commitment of each member. Finally, large boards tend to have numerous committees. These committees do not exist because they help the board govern effectively, they exist simply to guarantee that every board member serves on one. This excess baggage is structural inefficiency at its worst.

If large boards are generally not the way to go, what about really small ones, those with fewer than ten members? They promise more streamlined functioning due to increased focus and less effort required to communicate with the board and to coordinate its activities. Also, smaller boards tend to be more functionally flexible.

However, boards with ten or fewer members have several significant disadvantages. First, one or two members can dominate a board and exert disproportionate influence. Second, such small boards often fail to develop a positive group dynamic because they lack an appropriate mix of skills, knowledge, and experience. Third, the unplanned departure of one or two members can disrupt the board due to lack of bench strength. Finally, such boards often demand too much of their members through multiple committee assignments and consequently run the risk of burnout.

While each health care organization may have unique circumstances and requirements, the most efficient board size is typically no fewer than ten and no more than twenty members. Additionally, we suggest that boards be composed of an odd number of members, to preclude the possibility of tie votes on controversial issues.

The ideal board (with thirteen, fifteen, or seventeen members) is small enough to function as an effective deliberative body without the need for an overly active, dominant executive committee. It is also large enough to create cohesive teams with an appropriate mix of skills, experience, and other desired characteristics. A board in this size range is large enough to shoulder necessary governance responsibilities and roles, and also to function unimpeded by the absence of several members from meetings.

Board size may vary among different boards within a system or multiple-governance organization. Some systems will allow subsidiary boards to grow to a larger size (twenty members or more) while keeping the parent board in the smaller size range (thirteen to fifteen members). The rationale for doing this is that the larger subsidiary boards allow for more involvement of community members and key stakeholder groups.

While this rationale may make some sense, it is important to remember that subsidiary boards (unless they are purely advisory bodies) are governing entities. They have important functions to perform and legal duties to fulfill. Consequently, they should be structured primarily for effectiveness. We have seen many systems limit board size to a recommended range of thirteen to fifteen members for all their boards, and feel that this approach has merit.

Committee Structure

One of the most important yet most neglected structural issues in governance is the relationship of boards to their committees. Some boards function without committees, as a so-called committee of the whole. However, the vast majority use committees to assist them in their work.

A key concept of the board-committee relationship is that committees should support and advance the work of the board, and the board should control and coordinate its committees. In many organizations, the reverse is unfortunately true. If a board does not control its committees, it will be controlled by them. With various committees pulling in different directions, attempting to advance different agendas, and focusing on wildly different levels of detail, it is almost impossible for a board to govern effectively and efficiently.

Committees cannot be expected to perform the work of the full board—and should never be allowed to do so. With the exception of an executive committee, committees should not formulate policy or make decisions—that is, they should not discharge the board's responsibilities. Rather, they should perform staff work related to governance and make recommendations to the full board.

Given the number and magnitude of issues that most health care organization boards face today, as well as the volume of work they must accomplish, we believe a well-structured and tightly controlled small group of committees is critical to high levels of governance performance and contributions.

The basic questions that every board should routinely ask itself are: What committees, if any, should we have? What should these committees do? Most boards do not address these questions; they have a standing committee structure that does not change from year to year. This rigid structure carries the risk of freezing the focus and work of a board so that it cannot adapt to changing circumstances.

Boards often struggle to address new issues with an old, increasingly outmoded committee structure. As the incongruity grows, boards tend to fall into one of three traps. First, they assign new topics to existing committees whose focus or charge addresses issues of past importance (for example, assigning the issue of community health assessment to a board quality improvement committee that focuses on inpatient quality). Here, it is common for the committee to continue to focus on its original assignment because of its established expertise and comfort level, and neglect the important new assignment. Second, they create new committees to address new issues while continuing to maintain the old committees as well.

This results in too many committees, and a two-class committee structure with important (new) and unimportant (old) committees consuming excessive board and management time. Third, they leave the old committee structure alone and address new issues through the formation of ad hoc committees or task forces. This approach can soon grow out of hand and create a Byzantine, top-heavy committee structure causing governance gridlock.

These common pitfalls of board-committee structure and functioning should be avoided. The question is how to do this and have a functional, efficient committee structure that is relevant to current and emerging issues in addition to board responsibilities and roles. The approach we recommend is for each board to tailor its committee structure and functioning to the established priorities of the board. This can be accomplished through the use of a "zero-based" board committee structure (Orlikoff and Totten, 1996).

The Zero-Based Approach

A zero-based committee structure forces a board to seriously reevaluate its committee structure and functioning every year. A board ends each fiscal year with the dissolution of its standing committees—a blank slate. The board must then determine which, if any, of the previous committees should continue to exist, and whether new ones should be created.

We believe that only when the specific focus and function of a board has been defined can that board appropriately consider the issue of what committees it should have. Once the board gains this focus through the development of annual board goals and objectives (a concept addressed in Chapter Eight), it can then create its committee structure for the coming year accordingly.

Boards that use a zero-based approach usually find that several committees do carry over from year to year. These are the committees that support the execution of core board responsibilities. Even so, much of the value of zero-based design is that it forces the board to critically and explicitly assess each committee, taking none for granted. Every committee from the previous year is evaluated based on its relevance to current organizational needs and strategy, board goals and objectives for the coming year, and the board's responsibilities. This exercise usually results in a modification of the previous committee structure, as well as a change in the charge, focus, and work plans for those committees that are retained. The zero-based committee design process is a powerful form of continuous governance improvement.

Illustration: Zero-Based Committee Design

If, for example, an organization decides to identify a partner with needed strengths and merge with it, and the board incorporates this strategy into its goals and objectives, it might create a merger and affiliation committee. The life of this committee would most likely correspond to the length of the merger process and the need for a level of board involvement that could best be supported by such a committee. At the end of the year when the merger takes place, the board disbands the committee rather than keeping it around in case another merger comes up in the future. Here, the board has tailored its committee structure and focus to the strategy of the organization and its own goals and objectives.

When specific committees are mandated in the by-laws, any change in committee structure requires an amendment of them. There is an understandable reluctance to revise by-laws annually, and so we suggest that they be amended to incorporate the zero-based design process that will be followed each year. The by-laws simply state that the board specifies its standing committees at the beginning of each fiscal year, and that these committees cease to exist at the end of the year.

Core Board Committee Structure and Function

Even with the use of the zero-based design process, certain board committees will probably continue from year to year. Such core committees are necessary because board meetings are usually too brief to allow a board to adequately perform all of its work. Additionally, certain aspects of a board's work can be better addressed by smaller groups that are carefully composed to include individuals with specific talents or qualifications who are not board members.

A key structural challenge facing every health care organization board is how to subdivide governance work among committees in a way that facilitates effectiveness but does not compromise the accountability and integrity of the full board.

First, boards should employ the zero-based design process. Second, the process itself should be guided by four principles.

Authority: The full board bears ultimate responsibility for governing the organization. Board committees, except in very carefully specified and infrequent situations (such as an executive committee that can act in defined emergency situations), do not have any independent authority to act on behalf of the full board.

Minimalism: The smallest possible number of board committees should be created in any given year.

Structure: Committees should be structured for the primary purpose of helping the board fulfill its responsibilities and roles.

Charter: The board should control the work of each committee through the use of committee charters and annual work plans (addressed further in Chapter Eight).

A good starting point for core board committees is the set of governance responsibilities discussed in Chapter Four: ends, management performance, quality, finance, and self-management. This is not to say that a board must have these five committees, but it is a useful point of departure. For example, a board may combine two of these responsibilities into one committee; management performance and self-management commonly go together. Or a board may decide that one or more of the responsibilities should be fulfilled by the board as a whole.

Employing governance responsibilities as a design template will often result in some combination of the following as a board's core committees:

- *Planning Committee* (a misnomer, in terms of focus and functioning). This is the committee on ends; it assists the board in fulfilling its responsibility for formulating an organization's vision and goals.

- *Finance Committee*. Perhaps the most common of all board committees, it assists the board in fulfilling its responsibility for enhancing the organization's long-term financial viability. It does this by specifying financial objectives, ensuring that financial plans are crafted by management, and monitoring and assessing financial performance.

- *Quality and Community Health Committee*. Assists the board in enhancing the quality of care, including improving the health of the communities served, monitoring and evaluating the process and outcomes of care, and credentialing physicians and other professional clinical staff.

- *Governance Committee*. Assists the board in ensuring its own effective and efficient performance, including the nominating, board self-evaluation, and governance education processes.

- *Executive Committee*. Assists the board in emergency situations requiring action where it is impossible to

convene a full board meeting. Frequently, this committee will also assist the board by taking the lead in executive management performance improvement, CEO
evaluation, board goal and objective setting, and board
agenda planning. This is typically the only committee
that is, in limited and defined situations, empowered to
act with the authority of the full board.

Appendix B presents sample board committee descriptions and
charges.

Committee Structure in Multiple-Governance Entities

The issue of the relationship of a board to its committees is challenging enough in a single-board organization, and it can become
incredibly complex when there are multiple boards to coordinate.
The organization must deal with a variety of questions: Should each
board in the system have committees? Should subsidiary boards
determine their committee structure and functioning or should this
be done by the parent? Should subsidiary boards report to the parent directly or through its committees?

Since our bias is toward streamlined governance, we believe the
principle of minimalism should be applied to the number of board
committees as well as the number of boards.

In decentralized governance structures, or modified centralized
structures, it is common to find committees for each subsidiary
board as illustrated in Exhibit 6.11. Frequently, these board committees come in matched sets, duplicated over and over for each
board.

We strongly recommend against duplicative board committees in
a multiple-governance entity. Duplication usually creates far too many
committees, consuming excessive amounts of executive management
and board time and blurring distinctions in governance responsibilities and roles between the multiple boards. Governance gridlock is
the usual result—often degenerating into outright conflict.

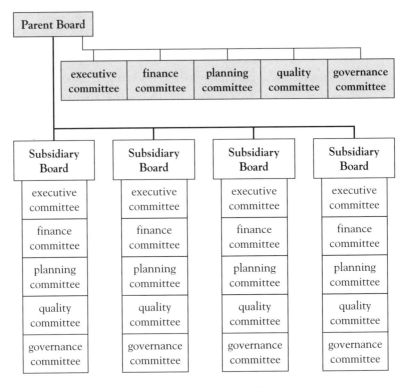

Exhibit 6.11. Duplicative Board Committee Structure

We recommend that board committees be centralized under the parent board, and that as a general rule, subsidiary boards be severely limited as to the number (if any) and type they have. Further, before any subsidiary board committee is created or allowed to continue into a coming year, the need for its existence must be questioned and its work clearly defined and limited relative to other boards and committees in the system. Consider the following example.

Illustration: Multiplying Meetings

Imagine a system with one parent and six subsidiary boards. That is seven governance entities. If the parent board has five committees and the subsidiary boards have none, that's twelve governance entities. Now imagine this system also has duplicative board committees, with the parent having five committees and each subsidiary having five committees. Now we have forty-two governance entities! Putting aside functionality for a second, if each meets monthly, we have a system that must staff and support, and board members who must prepare for and attend, *504 meetings per year!* We are hard-pressed to conceive of many situations where more than forty governance entities and five hundred meetings per year will add value to a health care organization.

A system employing a decentralized structure has a subsidiary board govern a hospital. The two responsibilities assigned to the subordinate board are financial oversight and assuring quality and credentialing of medical staff. Should the hospital board have its own finance and quality and credentialing committees?

The answer to this question partially depends on the structural model employed. In other words, if the system has chosen a decentralized, organization-based model of governance, it would probably also choose a duplicative board committee structure. (That's another reason we dislike the organization-based model!) A system with a modified centralized, functional model of governance would probably choose to centralize most committees under the parent board, and create subsidiary board committees only as necessary to support specific functions.

In most cases, we think the answer to the question of whether the subsidiary board should have its own committees should be no, even in the decentralized, organization-based model. Here, the subsidiary board has only two responsibilities: finance and quality. Both of these are limited in scope. Cannot this board most efficiently perform the work required as a committee of the whole? We think so.

Clearly, this issue is complicated by how and how much governance work is subdivided among boards in a system. The more work a subsidiary board has, the more the argument can be made that it may need committees of its own. The issue of subsidiary board committees is a reflection of the structural governance model chosen, as well as the way governance responsibilities are subdivided within the system.

Committee Reporting Relationships

Should subsidiary boards report to the parent board directly or through its committees? This is an issue where structure and function intersect.

Our approach again rests on the four principles outlined earlier (authority, minimalism, structure, and charter). We believe the best approach is for subsidiary boards to report through the parent's committees.

For example, suppose a parent board has a finance committee. Further, suppose that there are three subsidiary boards in the system, each responsible for monitoring the finances of their organizations (or regions, or functions) consistent with the budget approved by the parent board. These subsidiary boards are also charged with the responsibility of ensuring that their organizations accomplish financial goals and objectives established by the system board. What should the reporting relationship be regarding finance?

We believe that the subsidiary boards should be accountable to the parent's finance committee. Further, part of the charter and work plan of the parent board's finance committee should be to coordinate the financial activities of the subsidiary boards and monitor their performance. In this arrangement, parent board committees become funnel points for coordinating and overseeing the activities of subsidiary boards with respect to specific delegated responsibilities.

The Board–Executive Committee Relationship

Perhaps the most important but most unexamined board-committee relationship is the relationship of the board to its executive committee. The executive committee is empowered to act with the full authority of the board. Therefore, defining its role in relation to that of the board is absolutely crucial to effective and efficient governance.

Why do executive committees exist? They are a vestige of the era of large boards. In a large board, an executive committee often functioned as the real board; discharging most governance responsibilities and roles. In many of these situations, the full board became simply a rubber stamp of executive committee actions. This dominant executive committee–weak board arrangement can still be found in some health care organizations today.

A dominant executive committee is one that is invested with (or assumes) the authority to take broad action without approval from the full board, and one that makes frequent use of this authority. This arrangement is diametrically opposed to effective governance. A dominant executive committee usually results not just in ineffective governance but in dysfunctional governance. This results from the negative dynamic that inevitably emerges from the two-class governance system caused by a dominant executive committee.

It may seem efficient to have a dominant executive committee, but the practice only builds up trouble among the second-class board members—that is, everybody who isn't on the committee. People who serve as directors and bear the risks of directors without having genuine influence over their organization become increasingly frustrated and angry with their lack of involvement in key issues and their limited authority. This anger soon becomes focused at the executive committee and its members. The board attempts to wrest power, information, and control from the executive committee. The executive committee, in response, becomes even more authoritarian and secretive. Things continue to boil until open conflict results. Sometimes the board resigns, sometimes the board is able to reconstitute the executive committee and restrict its authority. Often, nothing conclusive happens to resolve the conflict, which simmers below the surface, erupting at particularly inopportune moments. Such a negative dynamic is a major—and almost insurmountable—barrier to effective governance.

There are, however, valid reasons to have executive committees. Perhaps the most compelling reason is to provide for rapid response in emergency situations that require board action where it is impossible to convene a quorum of the full board. Since these situations are rare (especially in the context of smaller boards, monthly board meetings, and emergency meetings by conference call), executive committee actions should be equally rare.

In addition to emergency authority, an executive committee can also be assigned other critical tasks:

CEO *performance evaluation:* Here, the executive committee takes the lead with regard to CEO performance objectives, evaluation, and compensation, and makes recommendations to the board. The board, however, makes all decisions.

Governance improvement: The core governance responsibility for self-management includes oversight of board self-evaluation, continuing education, and new board member recruitment and orientation.

Board agenda planning: Consistent with board-approved annual goals and objectives, the executive committee can plan agendas for board meetings.

In smaller boards that meet frequently, have low quorum requirements, and permit telephonic meetings, an executive committee may be entirely unnecessary. For larger boards, or those that meet infrequently or have high quorum requirements or prohibit telephonic meetings, an executive committee can help ensure that board action is taken when necessary. However, the role, function, authority, and very need for an executive committee should be reviewed annually as part of the zero-based committee design process.

The proper role of an executive committee is not to control a board but to support it. To ensure this, a board must define and limit the authority of its executive committee, retain such authority as necessary to prevent a dominant committee from emerging, and annually define its charge and scope of responsibilities.

Principles of Effective Structure

As the twists and turns of this chapter indicate, governance structure is a complex topic. Some boards interpret this as a reason for neglect; it is easy to not think about governance structure. Health care organizations that do not think about it, however, tend to create Byzantine governance structures that compromise governance performance and contributions.

Many will say, "We have many of the characteristics of governance structure that you advise against, and it hasn't hurt us at all." This may be true, but it is also true that when the predictable negative consequences of bad governance structure become manifest, it is usually at a time of crisis. In other words, when bad structures contribute to bad governance, it is often at the precise time when effective governance is needed most.

While appropriate governance structure will be tailored to the specific circumstances of individual health care organizations, there are common principles of efficient structures:

- *Intentionality*. Governance structure is planned and is based on conscious, explicit choices. It is not simply allowed to evolve, nor is it justified by such statements as "we've always done it this way."

- *Functionality*. The primary purpose of structure is to facilitate effective governance.

- *Evaluation*. Governance structure is evaluated annually. It is fine-tuned on an ongoing basis, and significantly modified when necessary.

- *Simplicity*. The fewer governance entities, the better.

Statement	No	Somewhat	Yes
• My organization has too many boards.	3	2	1
• The governance structure of my organization is based on a carefully thought-out and explicit design process—it did not evolve by chance and circumstance.	1	2	3
• We have conducted a thorough review and assessment of my organization's board structure in the last two years.	1	2	3
• My board is the right size, having between ten and twenty members.	1	2	3
• The number and type of committees facilitates my board's ability to discharge its responsibilities and roles, in addition to meeting new challenges as they arise.	1	2	3
• Each board committee has a charter that clearly specifies its objectives and tasks.	1	2	3

(continued on page 149)

- *Consistency.* The governance structure is consistent with management and clinical structures. For example, a three-hospital system with centralized management and a single medical staff should have a centralized or modified centralized governance structure.

Structure is a delicate latticework of related factors, each of which has a critical and highly interdependent impact on governance performance and contributions. Structure, however, does not create function; it can only facilitate or inhibit it.

Statement	No	Somewhat	Yes
• Committees do not usurp the responsibilities or authority of the full board.	1	2	3
• My board engages in a zero-based committee design process each year.	1	2	3
TOTAL =			

Governance Check-Up: Structure
Source: © Orlikoff and Associates, Inc., 1998.

```
8        10      12      14      16      18      20      22      24
|_____|_____|_____|_____|_____|_____|_____|_____|

Low                     Moderate                       High
Performance             Performance                    Performance
```

Benchmark Practices: Structure

• Make certain that management and clinical structures are consistent with governance structure. It doesn't make sense to have incompatible leadership structures, such as centralized management and decentralized governance.

• Review your current governance structure. How many boards are there in your organization? Are there clear organizing principles for your current governance structure? If so, what are they? If not, what implicit principles are suggested by your structure?

• Determine your organization's model of governance structure. Is it centralized, decentralized, or modified centralized? If your organization has subordinate boards, how are they organized (organizationally, regionally, or functionally, or a combination)?

• Know your governance structure. Have a governance organization chart developed, one that outlines all the boards and board committees in your organization, as well as their reporting relationships. Have this chart placed in the board policy book and in the front section of every board agenda book for easy and frequent reference.

- Review the size of your board. How many members currently serve on your board? How many board members do the by-laws stipulate? If there is a difference in these two numbers, what is the reason for it? Is the actual board size appropriate, or is the board too large or too small? Why is your board the size that it is? Should the size of your board be modified, and if so, how?

- During your next board meeting, look around the board table. Do you know who everyone is? If not, your board may be too large.

- Review the committee structure of your board. Ask each board member to answer the question: How many committees of the board are there?

- Ensure that every board committee has a charter that clearly outlines its scope of work.

- Avoid duplicative board committees if your organization has multiple boards. Subsidiary boards should not have the same committees as the parent does.

- Use the zero-based committee design process. Evaluate your board's committee structure every year and modify it as necessary based on organizational need and strategy as well as board focus and priority.

7

Governance Composition

A film student approached famous film director John Houston and challenged: "Are you aware that at least 50 percent of the success of your films is simply due to casting?" Mr. Houston is said to have replied, "Dear boy, my films are 100 percent casting!"

Whether the story is true or not, the fact is Houston had a deep understanding that casting decisions—choosing who plays in the various roles of a film—are critical to that film's success. This same principle is also true for boards.

Pause and Reflect: Your Board's Cast

Is your board's composition different today from what it was five years ago? If so, how?

What restrictions or requirements, if any, are placed on the composition of your board? For example, are any ex officio positions mandated in the by-laws? Do any external groups appoint or elect members to your board? Is your board required to have a certain percentage or number of its members drawn from defined groups or geographic areas?

Why do you think you were selected as a board member?

Is the current composition of your board ideal? If so, why? If not, why not?

We turn now to the topic of board composition and address such issues as the selection and recruitment of new members, reappointment of members to additional terms, terms and term limits, and the removal of nonperforming members from office. How and why the members of a board are chosen—and how their skills, qualifications, experience, and backgrounds are balanced and blended—has a monumental impact on governance performance and contributions.

Casting Basics

No other characteristic so directly and immediately affects the performance and contributions of a board as its makeup. Accordingly, members should be chosen with great care. This care should not just be taken in the selection of individual members, but should be invested in creating a criteria-based process for designing the board's composition. This process should take into account the needs of the board, its strengths and weaknesses, the likely contributions of potential members, and the current balance of skills, experience, and other competencies.

We are often asked, "Who should be on our board?" Our response is, "Well, tell us what your board does, the key issues it will be facing, its focus for the coming year." This often draws blank stares, or the challenge, "What does that have to do with who is on the board?" Of course, it has everything to do with it!

Many boards fail to recognize that it is impossible to develop an effective process for board composition before they have clearly conceptualized their responsibilities and roles. If you don't know what you're supposed to do, how can you tell who's got what it takes to help you do it? The questions should flow in this order: What is our board supposed to do? Once this is clarified, the question becomes: What individual skills, characteristics, and backgrounds of members are needed for the board to effectively do what it is supposed to? Health care organization boards face a variety of different issues, some explicit, some implicit. Each issue may create different and often incompatible demands with respect to composition.

A common example of the tension created by the need for different board member capacities and competencies is the issue of community representation and business skill (community representation is discussed in greater detail in a later section). If an objective of a board is to "represent the community," this calls for a membership composed of a cross-section of the community. Yet if the board is supposed to govern the organization with business acumen, that calls for members with significant business expertise. So, should this board emphasize community representation over business acumen or vice versa? Should half of the board be selected as community representatives and the other half as business experts? Should only people who both represent different components of the community and have business expertise be allowed to serve on the board?

Such questions are challenging enough for any board, yet they represent only two sets of characteristics and qualifications for potential board members. Consider how the issue is compounded when other board member skills and qualifications are desired—specialized health care or insurance expertise that cannot be obtained in the local community, membership in key constituencies (physician groups or sponsoring religious orders or subordinate organization boards or purchasers of the organization's services), legal expertise, political contacts, philanthropic contacts, wealth, past board experience. . . . The list is endless, and you will never find all the potentially desirable characteristics combined in a single individual.

There is tremendous variation in the sophistication of health care organization boards throughout the country. There is often as much variation in the sophistication, dedication, and performance of the individual board members. The former is partially due to the wide variation in the definition of governance responsibilities and roles among boards. The variation in quality from member to member within a board is largely due to a lack of meaningful selection, evaluation, and reappointment processes.

The best way of ensuring that board members are up to the task of governing complex health care organizations is to use a criteria-based selection and reappointment process—a board member credentialing process. As was discussed in Chapter Four, physicians are subject to credentialing to be appointed and reappointed to a medical staff. Board members should be credentialed as well, even though no outside agency provides licensing. Such a process should be based on very explicit and carefully developed criteria.

Initial Selection

There are any number of possible criteria to identify and evaluate candidates for board membership, as well as to evaluate current members who are up for renewal of their terms. According to the American Hospital Association and Ernst & Young, these were the top selection criteria for hospital board membership in 1997:

1. Values consistent with hospital

(tied with)

1. Community leadership

2. Financial and business acumen

3. Strategic planning and visioning

4. Time availability

5. Political influence

We see the growing use of past governance experience as one criterion to evaluate prospective board members. Particularly in large integrated delivery systems, board members are frequently sought who already have some type of governance experience, whether within the system on a subsidiary board, on other health care boards, or on any type of nonprofit or commercial board.

While any of these criteria may have value, we believe that rather than focus on any one criterion, or on a handful of them (everyone has a favorite), it is essential to develop a process that uses categories of weighted criteria. In this way, and using the board profiling process discussed in the next section, a logical and relatively objective method can be used to compose a board and balance member competencies and capacities.

There are a number of ways to group the criteria that can be employed to select board members. We find it useful to think in terms of general qualifications criteria, demographic criteria, specific qualifications criteria, and position criteria. These four categories are fairly inclusive, but we do not regard it as important that an organization use this list—or the sample criteria—as given. What is important is that every board explicitly develops its own list. The actual criteria chosen by any board will vary depending on many variables, not the least of which is the type of organization; a parent board might use different criteria from those used by a hospital or medical group board. The overall categories and the sample lists presented in this section derive from the work of Orlikoff and Totten (1995).

General Qualifications

These are criteria that all board members must meet. They should be rigidly applied to all prospective board members. For example, what value is there in putting on the board a skilled, intelligent, well-qualified individual who cannot attend a majority of board and committee meetings, cannot accept the board's style of decision making, or cannot keep confidential matters confidential?

Typical general qualifications criteria:

- Willingness to serve on the board

- Ability to meet the projected time commitment (attendance at board meetings, committee meetings, retreats, in addition to preparation)

- Capacity for attention to this organization (does not sit on more than three other boards if currently employed, or on six other boards if retired or not employed on a full-time basis)

- Ability to function as a member of a deliberative body (to participate in group decision making using preestablished principles of the group and ability to support board decisions even when the individual voted against the majority)

- Willingness to participate in board orientation and continuing education (time commitment to initial orientation process, attendance at a defined number of educational events per term, as well as regularly reading health care and governance books and articles provided by the organization)

- Objectivity

- Intelligence

- Communication skills

- Integrity and the absence of serious conflicts of interest

- Ideology and values consistent with those of the organization

Demographics

These criteria relate to issues such as the geographic location of board members, community involvement or representation, as well as age, gender, and ethnicity. This category of criteria, as opposed to the general qualification criteria, are typically applied more as flexible guidelines to achieve some desired mix of member characteristics.

Typical demographic selection criteria:

- Certain percentage of members reside within communities served by the organization (something we suggest boards employ as a guideline rather than a requirement)

- At least one member serving on the board does not live in the organization's service area

- Age parameters for board membership—a minimum age of twenty-one and a maximum of seventy-five

- Membership balance based on gender

- Membership balance based on race and ethnicity

- Membership balance based on socioeconomic status reflective of communities served

- Minimum education level requirement

Specific Qualifications

This category reflects both the ongoing and specific needs of the board and those of the organization being governed. Specific qualifications criteria may address the knowledge, skills, experience, occupation, contacts, politics, affluence, and other desired characteristics of members. Specific criteria are typically variably applied to select members with different but complementary skill sets and experience. It is through the variable use of this and other categories of criteria that a board is able to avoid becoming an inbred, homogenous group by creating a blended mix of skills, experience, and knowledge among its members.

Typical specific qualifications criteria:

- Past experience on other boards (such as experience as a health care organization board member or on the board of a large private sector corporation or nonprofit organization)

- Professional and business achievement

- Membership balance based on specific occupations and skills, such as in business, medicine, law, nursing, or others

- Demonstrated leadership skills

- Demonstrated big picture thinking ability

- Demonstrated systems thinking capacity

- Demonstrated record of community involvement and commitment

- Political involvement or connections

- Competencies aligned with the strategy and needs of the organization (such as experience in mergers, down-sizing, reengineering in other organizations, integrating new business ventures into existing ones, or industries that have undergone major systemic change)

- One executive or board member of a major purchaser of the organization's services

- Professional experience in clinical health care

- Professional experience in health care administration

Position

Many boards establish seats for individuals who hold specific jobs, usually within the organization. Position criteria identify all individuals who will be ex officio members. A very common example of such criteria is found in the by-laws of many hospitals, which require that the CEO and the chief of the medical staff be granted ex officio board membership with vote.

Positions typically considered for ex officio status:

- CEO of organization

- Other health care organization senior executives

- Chief of the medical staff

- President of a strategically critical physician organization

- Chair of the foundation

- President of the auxiliary

- Designated representative of sponsoring religious order

- Designated representatives of the two parent corporations in a joint venture board

(*Note:* Although we list many different possible position criteria, as a general rule we recommend that no more than two individuals serve on a board at any one time in an ex officio capacity.)

Term Renewal

All boards should have an explicit policy that term renewal is not automatic! All board members should be subject to an evaluation at the conclusion of each term to determine if their performance— as well as the anticipated needs of the board—warrant their reappointment. This is an important point, and it emphasizes effective board composition as an ongoing process. Even if a board member has performed well, reappointment to another term may not be in the board's interest. Why? Because board composition needs may have changed due to significant alteration in strategy, market conditions, business activities, or organizational partners. Such a board might find that the current member's skills are no longer as critical as they once were, and that the board could be better served by bringing on individuals with skill sets more compatible with emerg-ing needs. The outgoing member should be apprised of this, thanked for the service, and given appropriate recognition.

Board member term renewal thus has two components—com-paring the skills of the member to the needs of the board as dis-cussed earlier, and evaluating the performance of the member during the past term. To conduct this performance evaluation, we suggest two basic categories of criteria: board member citizenship and board member performance.

Board Member Citizenship

Board member citizenship criteria relate to the necessary attributes of effective boardsmanship. Has the individual done the things board members have a right to expect of each other?

Typical citizenship criteria:

- Board meeting attendance requirement met

- Board committee meeting attendance requirement met

- Continuing education requirement met

- Attended annual board retreat

- Attended defined number of medical staff or physician organization meetings and committee meetings

- Attended minimum number of social events where board member presence was requested

Board Member Performance

Board member performance criteria relate to activities and attrib-utes that directly affect the board's ability to discharge its responsi-bilities and roles. Has the individual worked smoothly with the board and done his or her share, without creating unnecessary work or stress for others?

Typical performance criteria:

- Active and thoughtful contributor at board and committee meetings

- Does not attempt to dominate discussion at meetings

- Reads agenda materials prior to meetings and comes prepared to address the defined issues

- Supports board actions and does not attempt to subvert past decisions or policy

- Is comfortable expressing a dissenting opinion or vote

- Expresses dissenting opinion constructively, not in a negative or ad hominem manner

- Integrates continuing education into board deliberation and function

- Has not violated confidentiality of boardroom

- Has not violated conflict-of-interest policy

- Clearly places the best interests of the organization above personal or business interests

- Understands and abides by policies and procedures governing board member conduct

- Supports the organization's vision and mission

- Is well versed in the strategy of the organization, and uses it as the basis for deliberating and considering issues before the board

- Has communicated effectively with key constituents regarding board positions when asked to do so

Applying the Criteria

Clearly, the evaluation of individual members who are up for renewal of their terms is a delicate exercise. There is typically great concern that those members whose performance is being evaluated should not be offended. (A certain amount of delicacy is natural here. After all, the sitting directors are vividly clear on the point that it will be their turn to be evaluated soon!) Unfortunately, this often translates into some members being reappointed when it would have been best for the board if they had taken their leave.

Effective boards govern based on a culture of performance and accountability—on principle, not personality. A significant part of such a culture is the clear understanding, driven by explicit policy, that the performance of every member will be evaluated based on established criteria as well as on the continued relevance of the member's skills and experience to the organization's and the board's needs. Further, it is understood that the purpose of board membership is not to benefit, protect, or aggrandize the individual member; it is to benefit the organization and its stakeholders.

Once this principle is adopted by a board, then it can establish a meaningful and fair process of member performance evaluation. This should involve the board's assigning responsibility for the process to a committee (for example, executive, nominating, or governance). This committee should develop a draft set of evaluation criteria, such as those suggested earlier, along with weightings for each criterion. Some criteria will be much more important than others. Once the weighted criteria are approved by the board, the committee is charged with conducting the evaluations. This consists of comparing the criteria to the member's performance, and making a recommendation to the board consistent with the profile. The committee is further charged with assessing the criteria and the relative weightings annually and recommending appropriate modifications.

One significant problem with the evaluation of member performance is that, for the vast majority of boards, the evaluation is subjective; members have no idea how their performance will be assessed. Having a set of explicit criteria that are weighted in terms of their relative importance makes the evaluation process much more palatable to all involved. Because errant members know the criteria and further know that they have not met several crucial ones, they also know they are not likely to be reappointed—and they often refrain from seeking another term, which saves face for everyone. Furthermore, performance criteria also tend to stimulate better performance as members strive to meet the explicit expectations.

Board Profiling

The development and use of criteria for the identification and selection of new members and evaluation of current members for term renewal helps build better boards. But the independent use of a criteria-based process can still result in a homogenous board lacking critical skills or other necessary characteristics. The best board composition results are achieved when the criteria-based process is used in tandem with board profiling.

Board profiling consists of developing a chart that outlines the skills, qualifications, demographic characteristics, and tenure of every current member. Exhibit 7.1 provides an illustration.

Once developed, the profile provides a detailed and comprehensive map of a board's composition and aids in identifying member competency and capacity gaps and redundancies. Profiling might result in certain criteria being given a higher priority than others, new criteria being created, and old criteria being modified or eliminated. It is the dynamic interplay between the current board profile and the criteria that creates the process that best contributes to effective and constantly evolving board composition.

Pause and Reflect: Board Profiling

Develop a quick profile of your board. For each board member, list special expertise, areas of interest, professional background, type and length of community involvement, age, residency, sex, race,

Board Members

Criteria	John Heilgest	Nancy Stewart	Ralph Cortez	Sr. Kyle McCarthy	Dr. John Winters
age	52	63	37	74	58
sex	male	female	male	female	male
race or ethnicity	black	white	Latino	white	white
residence	inside service area	inside service area	inside service area	outside service area	outside service area
occupation	CEO Capstad, Inc.	homemaker	CEO, Quest Foundation	member Sr. of St. Joseph	physician (internist)
governance experience	high	low	medium	high	low
industry and market knowledge	medium	low	medium	high	low
clinical expertise	none	medium (former RN)	none	none	high (physician)
financial knowledge	high	low	high	low	low
management experience	high	low	high	none	none
experience with acquisitions and mergers	high	none	none	none	none
community and political contacts	some	great	great	none	none

Exhibit 7.1. Illustrative Board Profile

ethnicity, board tenure, and years remaining until the maximum term limit is reached. Now consider these questions:

Are there areas of duplication or clustering on the board? (For example, does your board have a majority of fifty-five-year-old white bankers who all live in the same community and have five years left until they reach the maximum term limit?) What characteristics, skills, and experiences are underrepresented on your board?

Based on the board profile, what key characteristics do you think are critical in the next three members recruited for the board?

Develop a profile of your ideal board necessary to help your organization achieve its key goals and fulfill its vision.

Compare the current board to your ideal profile. What differences exist? Based on these differences, what criteria for new member selection should your board develop and employ? What criteria for board member reappointment should be developed or discarded?

Once a board is comfortable with the accuracy of the profile of its current membership and its relationship to the modification of selection and evaluation criteria, a profile of the characteristics and composition of an ideal board can then be developed. The ideal is then compared to the current board profile to identify gaps. This can result in the refinement or development of new selection and evaluation criteria. Accordingly, a board is always selecting new members—and reappointing current ones to additional terms—in pursuit of an ideal composition.

Clearly, there is no one ideally composed board for all health care organizations. The ideal will be based on the circumstances confronting the organization and board needs, all of which change over time. The exercise of going through an annual process of updating the ideal profile helps a board keep these critical composition issues in the forefront of its thinking and planning.

Composition Models

The issue of who should be on a board is partially, or in some cases wholly, dependent on the model of composition employed (or, in some cases, mandated). There are three basic models: election, appointment, and self-perpetuation.

An *elected board* is one where members are selected by a vote of stakeholders. County, district, or public hospitals supported by tax dollars often have elected boards. Other examples can be found in hospitals and health systems that have a parent "corporator" model. Here, the corporators are usually community members who register or who pay a small one-time fee and thereby gain the authority to elect and remove board members. While this model provides some limited advantages, we do not believe they compensate for its significant disadvantages. Advantages include direct constituency control of the selection process and direct accountability of the board to its electorate. On the negative side, the elected board model typically results in boards that are composed of members who campaigned for office on specific agendas (no merger, more parking, no investment in outpatient surgery, a higher nurse-to-patient ratio). A politicized and divided board often results as various members focus on their specific agendas, neglecting other critical responsibilities. Further, these single-issue members usually filter most governance issues through their narrow frame of reference.

Usually, elected boards have very short terms of office, two years being typical. Without staggered terms there is the possibility of an entirely new board being elected every two years. With staggered terms, this board can still be disrupted with 50 percent turnover every year. The frequent turnover typical of elected boards contributes to lack of governance continuity. Another major drawback of elected boards is that they are usually prohibited from removing dysfunctional board members from office, as this authority rests with the electorate. So an elected board can have a director who is actively working against the strategy of the organization, who constantly violates the confidentiality of the boardroom, and who is in frequent conflict-of-interest situations, and the board can do nothing about it.

In an *appointed board* members are selected by some other entity; a parent board (in a system); parent or sponsor organization (in religious-sponsored systems and hospitals); or a governmental body (legislature, public health agency, county board of supervisors, or city council). The primary benefit of this model is the power it gives the appointing authority, who can ensure that all board members hold similar views and values and will work to advance specific— and hopefully shared—agendas. This model can work well if the appointing authority employs a logical, criteria-based process to identify, assess, and appoint members. If the appointing authority (like many we have seen) uses capricious, subjective criteria or hands out board appointments as political favors, a bad board will result. Another frequent drawback is that boards may be reluctant to make major decisions if they believe they are not in the best interests of the appointing authority or if they are uncertain of its position on the issue. This slows the decision-making process down as board members check all major decisions with the appointing authority. Finally, and perhaps most significantly, this model can blur responsibility as a result of confusion over who the real authority is: Is it the board, or is it the appointing authority? This is not always the case, especially in systems with multiple boards where the parent appoints the members of all subsidiary boards. Here, the ultimate authority is clear and appropriate: it rests with the parent.

The last model is the *self-perpetuating board*—so called because the board selects its own members and thus perpetuates itself. Here, a board will typically select its own members through a board election based on the nomination of a committee. This is the most common mechanism of new member selection in nonprofit health care organizations—and we also think it can be the best. Among its many advantages, it allows a board to control the continuity of its membership as well as the mix of skills and qualifications, to tailor the selection process to match changing conditions and needs, and to remove members from office when necessary to maintain integrity of board functioning. Finally, we have found this model to be the most flexible of the three. Of course, the self-perpetuating model can fail miserably and generate ineffective governance if not properly applied. Boards that use this model without an objective, criteria-based selection and term renewal process often become homogenous, inbred, and ineffective. Also, they can become isolated from the stakeholders they are supposed to serve. This creates the ultimate governance irony—a board that is responsible for acts that are contrary to the mission of the organization it governs. We believe these negatives can be avoided if a board resolutely uses an objective, criteria-based process to select and retain members.

Any single model or combination of the three models for board selection can be used in systems with multiple boards. For example, it is common for a parent board to use a self-perpetuating model, but employ appointment or election to compose subsidiary boards. (That is, the system board either surveys the field and selects appropriate members to appoint to the subsidiary board, or invites people to put themselves forward as candidates for election to it.) From the parent board's perspective, it is simply a self-perpetuating model, but from the subordinate boards' perspective, it is an appointed or elected model. We have also seen systems where all the parent board members are appointed by sponsoring religious orders, and the parent board then appoints or elects the members of all subsidiaries. In another variation, different models of determining composition can be employed for the same board. Here, the board may predominantly use a self-perpetuating model, but have a fixed percentage of its members appointed by an outside group, sponsoring religious order, or community organization. In our opinion, this model is workable as long as the board selects a majority of its own members.

Term Limits

Term limits refer to the maximum limitation on the number of consecutive terms, or years, board members can serve before they must step down. In the past, it was common for health care organization boards to have no term limits, and we still encounter board members who have served for twenty-five consecutive years! While such personal commitment is laudable, there is serious question as to whether it contributes to great governance.

Many argue that term limits are a terrible idea. They assert that term limits are arbitrary in the abstract and dangerous in practice, and that they force talented and valuable board members off the board—usually just when they are needed most. There is merit to these arguments. Term limits are arbitrary, and may indeed result in the loss of talented and dedicated board members. In a perfect world, we think term limits would be a terrible idea. Yet in this world, we recommend term limits wholeheartedly! Why? Simply because one of the hardest tasks for any board is to remove one of its own from office, or to not invite a board member back at the conclusion of a term. Firing a board member, especially a volunteer who is giving generous amounts of time, is a task that every board with which we have worked avoids like the plague.

Even if the errant board member is so weak or disruptive as to cause serious ongoing damage to board cohesiveness and effectiveness, most boards will not take action. The sad but inevitable cost of avoiding this unpleasant task is escalating governance dysfunction that inevitably hinders or harms the organization.

Term limits would be unnecessary—and the arguments against them would hold sway—if boards had the sort of meaningful member evaluation and board profiling processes discussed earlier in this chapter. These processes would produce a dispassionate assessment of the continued value of the individual to the board every time a term expired. Some board members would pass muster and continue to serve a large number of consecutive terms; others would not get past their first term.

We strongly recommend term limits as they provide a structured way to ensure turnover while preserving continuity, and are a powerful tool to help prevent boards from becoming stale and complacent. Additionally, in this challenging, hectic, uncertain health care environment, a limit on terms can be a blessing for individual board members. Dedicated volunteers who spend significant and ever-expanding amounts of time and energy—and who frequently put themselves at social and economic risk for their difficult decisions—are increasingly prone to burnout. Knowing that there is an end point to their service can help prevent this. Term limits can actually help get the best out of board members during their tenure.

We suggest some principles for the use of term limits. Term limits should neither be too short or too long. They must achieve a delicate balance between constantly revitalizing a board with new blood and maintaining continuity. They should be long enough to allow directors to learn their job, perform it well, and have the potential to rise to a position of leadership. They must be short enough to minimize the chance of board member burnout and to facilitate continual but gradual turnover.

Consistent with these principles, we recommend terms of three years, with a maximum limit of three consecutive terms, or a total of nine years. This "3–3" approach has several advantages. First, it takes a new member about three years to come up to speed and really learn the health care field, the organization, and the board's culture and its responsibilities and roles. This approach provides a new member with one term to come up to speed, an opportunity for a second term to make significant contributions to the board, and a possible third to ascend to a position of board leadership. Boards divided into three classes of staggered terms will never have more than one-third of their membership retire in any given year. Such boards usually have two-thirds of their membership with a minimum of three years of experience, and no more than one-third with less than three years.

To address the issue of arbitrary term limits' causing the loss of valuable talent, we recommend the following policy: upon reaching the term limit, a board member must withdraw from the board for a period of one year. At the conclusion of the year off, the individual can be invited back—once again eligible for three full terms. If the thought of losing such a fine individual for only a year is unacceptable, the individual can serve on a board committee for the one-year period. Term limits do not apply to any ex officio members. These individuals' tenure on the board is limited only by the duration of their position.

Finally, there are two issues relating to term limits for board officers. First, should a board member's maximum term limit be extended if they are elected board chair? We think the answer is yes, but the maximum extension should never exceed one term. In other words, even if board rules permit up to three 2-year terms as board chair, we do not recommend that an individual be allowed to serve a maximum of fifteen years (nine years as board member, then another six years as board chair). If a board member is elected board chair when they have one year left to serve on their third and final term, they should be allowed to serve out one complete two-year term as board chair. This would extend their tenure on the board one year past the stated term limit. Second, should there be term limits for board leaders? The answer is a definite yes! If term limits are appropriate for board members, they are certainly appropriate for board leaders. In addition, serving as board chair takes a significant amount of time and is a powerful position that, more than any other on the board, can exert huge influence on the function and effectiveness of a board. We recommend that terms for board chairs should be one year, or at most two years, with a maximum limit of two consecutive terms.

Removing a Board Member

One of the most distasteful tasks faced by a board is the occasional need to remove one of its own members from office in midterm. While never a pleasant task, it may unfortunately be a necessary one—and boards frequently find they do not have policy or process in place to address it properly. This common situation, coupled with the natural aversion to the issue, causes many boards to fail to take action when necessary.

An effective board creates a culture of performance and accountability, one that does not tolerate substandard performance by any member. Just as process and criteria are used for the selection of new members and the evaluation of their performance, so should they be used for the removal of members from office midterm.

Every board should have a by-law provision or policy that defines a mechanism for removing a member from office and prescribes criteria for when that mechanism must be used. Many boards have a vague clause in their by-laws that state a board member can be removed by a two-thirds majority vote of the board. Some of these by-law provisions state that the board member can be removed "for cause" or "for any reason." Here, the mechanism to remove a board member exists, but not the objective criteria for doing so. Just as criteria are necessary to an effective member evaluation process, they are necessary to a member removal process. Such criteria are best referred to in the by-laws but maintained in a separate board policy. This permits the continual revision and fine-tuning of the criteria without the need to revise the by-laws.

What actions or omissions are egregious enough to warrant a board member's removal from office? While each board must answer that question for itself, here are a few illustrations:

- Violating the conflict-of-interest policy

- Failing to attend a specified number of board meetings in a one-year period

- Failing to attend a specified number of consecutive board meetings

- Using information obtained as a board member in such a way as to derive personal financial benefit

- Violating the confidentiality policy

- Being verbally abusive to board members, physicians, or employees

- Making any physical assault on board members, physicians, or employees

- Working to subvert board policies or decisions

- Falling asleep on two or more occasions during board or board committee meetings

While some may disagree with our sample criteria and others may regard them with disbelief, let us emphasize that we have witnessed all of these behaviors. We stress, again: it is not important what we think the criteria should be. It is critical that a board debate this issue and specify its own criteria.

Just as with performance evaluation, developing a process and a set of criteria for removal of a member from office will go a long way toward preventing problems that would make it necessary to remove someone. Board members who know that violating the conflict-of-interest policy will bring about immediate termination from office are much less likely to do so. Members who cannot attend the minimum number of meetings will likely submit their resignations, or will rearrange their schedules to attend the meetings.

Frequently, subsidiary boards in systems do not have the authority to remove their own members from office; this authority typically rests with the parent. Here, the parent has the authority to remove members from its own board as well as from subsidiaries.

We recommend that parent boards adopt this philosophy: centralize authority but decentralize decision making. Consistent with this approach, many parent boards push down as many decisions and responsibilities to subordinate boards as possible This frees the system board to attend to big picture.

How then can a parent board control an empowered subsidiary board if it acts in a way inconsistent with directives and policy? The answer is found in the retained authority of the parent to remove any or all members from a subsidiary board at will. Many parent boards retain this authority, a so-called "doomsday button." The parent can remove an entire subsidiary board and then reconstitute it. The button would rarely be pushed, and then only under the most extreme circumstances. Having this authority, however, certainly does put the ultimate authority and control of subsidiary boards in the hands of the parent. It also allows a parent to empower subsidiary boards, assign them specific functions, and then step back and let them govern.

We recommend the doomsday button approach. It may rarely be used, but sends the clearest possible message of where ultimate authority lies. In addition, we recommend that the parent board develop criteria to remove individual subordinate board members for reasons of poor performance as discussed in the preceding section.

Ex Officio Members

Ex officio members are individuals who serve on a board by virtue of the position they hold. They can either be voting or nonvoting members. Normal term limits do not apply to such members, who serve as long as they are in the position that is granted board membership. An ex officio member of a board is usually a CEO, physician leader, or other health care professional or organizational insider.

Ex officio members are desirable, even essential, but we recommend there should not be more than two such members on a board at any given time. The value of having such insiders as voting members derives from the organizational and market-specific knowledge and experience they bring to a board.

If this is true, why only two ex officio board members? Why not more—or as many as possible? One or two ex officio members can provide valuable perspectives and expertise. More and there is a very real risk that a board will be dominated by insider perspectives and interests. This risk springs from the natural detachment of outsiders from the operations of the organization, and the intense involvement of insiders in the organization. Additionally, a maximum of two ex officio members ensures that a board has control of its own composition. The more ex officio positions on the board, the fewer at-large members can be chosen by the normal member selection process. As discussed earlier, the ability of a board to balance, blend, and constantly fine-tune its membership is key to governance effectiveness.

If a board has ex officio members, typically, one of these members will be the CEO of the organization or system.

CEO Board Membership

Should the CEO be an ex officio member of that organization's board? Our strong recommendation is yes. When the CEO sits on a board as a voting member, it emphasizes a key aspect of the unique relationship between the board and the CEO. This relationship is employer-employee but also a partnership. The CEO as a voting board member emphasizes the partnership aspect of the relationship and contributes to better governance.

Perspective: CEOs on Boards

A 1997 study by the American Hospital Association and Ernst & Young found that in hospitals, 46 percent of CEOs serve on the board with vote, 41 percent are ex officio members without vote, and 14 percent are either observers at or do not attend meetings. By

contrast, in systems 79 percent of system CEOs serve as voting
members of the board.

The notion that having the CEO on the board facilitates good
governance and better organizational performance is backed by
empirical evidence. A study of ninety California acute care hospitals showed that CEO participation on the board as a voting member significantly enhanced hospital performance (Molinari and
others, 1997). This study found that having the CEO as a voting
member of the board had more positive impact on effective governance and financial performance than did effective CEO contract
and performance evaluation procedures.

To a large degree, effective governance depends on the ability
of a board and CEO to work well together and to share power with
each other. When the CEO is a partner of the board, as evidenced
by board membership with vote, an effective working relationship
is facilitated. However, when the CEO is a passive observer at board
meetings, or worse still, is not even allowed to attend meetings, the
partnership aspect is diminished and the employer-employee relationship dominates. In such situations, a board deprives itself of
knowledge and experience that a CEO can and should bring to the
table.

We strongly recommend that the CEO not serve as the chair of
the board of a nonprofit health care organization.

There are those who argue that health care governance should
emulate commercial corporate governance, where the CEO often
also serves as board chair. We reject this argument on two counts.
First, when the CEO is also the board chair the distinction between
governance and management blurs, and the board-CEO relationship becomes ambiguous. Large amounts of power and authority
now rest with the CEO. This creates a significant imbalance of
power between the CEO and the board, and places the board in a
weak, passive posture. Second, the concept of effective governance

partly defined by a board that is not dominated by management insiders is spreading from the nonprofit health care sector to the commercial corporate sector. In fact, more corporate boards are abandoning the previously common practice of having the CEO serve as board chair, in addition to minimizing the number of insider board members ("The Best and Worst Boards," 1997).

Physician Board Membership

In addition to the CEO, it is also typical to have a physician leader as an ex officio board member. There are usually additional physicians who serve on health care organization boards who are not ex officio members, but are chosen by the regular board nomination process.

Physicians bring the same advantages as CEO membership on a board: professional expertise, an insider's view of the organization, operational experience, and demonstration of commitment to involve a key constituent group. In addition, some physicians also may bring another characteristic: representing a constituent group (physicians) that is key to the organization or system. It is this representational issue that poses a significant dilemma.

There are two types of physician members of a health care organization board: a physician member and a physician group representative. A *physician board member* is the same as any other member—chosen by the board's nomination and selection process, subject to term limits and performance evaluation, and not supposed to represent any interests other than what is best for the organization and its stakeholders. The *physician group representative* is different in that this individual is selected by a physician group, typically as its leader, and serves on the board as an ex officio member. The classic example of this is a hospital medical staff chief of staff, who serves on the board by virtue of holding that office and has the unique task of representing the medical staff interests. If the interests of the medical staff are inconsistent with those of other stakeholders, this representative is expected to advance the interests of the medical staff. Thus the primary loyalty of the physician representative is to the medical staff. Some argue that the physician representative is simply supposed to give voice to medical staff concerns, and then when it comes time to vote, he or she should do so reflecting the best interests of the organization and its stakeholders. This rarely happens in practice. In fact, we tend to see the reverse: not only does the physician group representative act in the best interests of the medical staff, but other physician board members do also.

What does a system board do for an ex officio physician leader? System boards, especially those with multiple hospitals and medical staffs, must rethink the notion of medical staff representation on the parent board and approach this issue from a systemic perspective. As a system grows, its hospitals diminish in importance as other components increase in importance. If the hospital diminishes in importance, so too does the hospital medical staff. Other physician groups that are specifically designed to link with the system to manage care and share financial risk increase in importance. Leaders of these groups (such as management service organizations, multispecialty group practices, independent practice associations, physician-hospital organizations, and physician organizations) may be more meaningful candidates for an ex officio position on the parent board.

How many physicians can a health care organization board have? IRS rules allow nonprofit boards to have up to 49 percent of their membership be "interested persons" (employees of the organization, such as the CEO, as well as any physicians who treat any patients in, do any business with, or derive any financial benefit from the organization). This 49 percent interested persons rule only applies if certain requirements are met. These requirements relate to ensuring that the organization operates for the benefit of the community and not the interested persons on the board. The first requirement is a strict conflict-of-interest policy. In addition, records must be maintained that demonstrate close adherence to the policy, including signed acknowledgments of the conflict-of-interest policy by each board member. The second requirement is the organization must conduct periodic reviews of all of its activities and operations, including those unrelated to its normal business, to ensure that it is conforming with its tax-exempt purposes. This review must ensure that the organization is not engaged in activities that provide inurement or unwarranted private benefit to the physicians or other interested board members.

Community Representation

Effective governance of nonprofit health care organizations involves the responsible stewardship of health resources to produce a sustained benefit to communities served. Conventional wisdom held that if governance was to truly benefit the community, it must be of the community; the board should be composed of members from the community served by the organization.

We believe that composing a board primarily to be representative of its community is a concept whose time has past. At a minimum, it is ripe for rigorous reexamination. Why? A single-minded focus on board composition based entirely on community representation may actually be antithetical to effective governance. The significant changes in the health care industry, affecting all organizations and their governance, challenge community-representational governance on many fronts.

The trend toward smaller boards presents fewer opportunities for community representation through fewer available seats. The growth in systems that serve large geographic areas makes equal community representation on a parent board impractical. Perhaps most significant, however, is the growing need for specific and scarce expertise and skill sets on health care boards. Many health care organizations, especially those in small communities and rural areas, may not be able to find the expertise they need close to home.

While it has been commonly assumed that there is a great value in having community members exclusively compose or dominate the boards of health care organizations, there has not been much attention given either to measuring the value or to weighing the tradeoffs. Is it possible for a board to govern a health care organization on behalf of a community without its members' being representative of that community? We believe the answer is yes.

Clearly, if potential members have both community involvement and necessary governance skills and expertise, this is a nonissue—go for both. But what about those situations where it is impossible to have both. Which characteristic is more important: community representation or specific expertise necessary to effective governance?

So we come again to the concept introduced at the beginning of this chapter: who should be on a board is a direct reflection of the board's purpose. If a board is supposed to be representative of its community, if this is its primary purpose, then representativeness is the most important selection criterion. If, however, boards have other and more important functions (as we believe most do), then other criteria become more important.

A board composed of individuals who do not live or work in the communities served by a health care organization can nevertheless be held accountable to those communities. Such a board can govern with its primary purpose being to provide benefit to the communities served.

As discussed in detail in Chapter Six and throughout this book, systems usually have multiple boards and serve many distinct communities. Consequently, it is difficult if not impossible for parent boards to be composed primarily on the basis of community representation. We find growing numbers of systems that are governed by focused, carefully composed boards with less than fifteen members. Increasingly, the members of such parent boards are not primarily chosen as community representatives. Large systems serve many communities, integrate many different businesses, and often have many local, subsidiary boards. At the same time, these parent boards face an ever more competitive environment that demands faster, more focused policy formulation and decision making. Such boards require skilled, tailored, professional expertise for maximum governance performance and contributions.

For these organizations, community representation through parent board membership is impractical to impossible. We believe that system board composition based primarily on community representation is a vestige of earlier, simpler times and is no longer appropriate. Furthermore, we suggest that system board composition based on community representation is likely to hinder the governance effectiveness necessary to lead the organization successfully into the future.

Local or subsidiary boards in a system, however, are a different story. Many are charged with a community liaison role. Consequently, there will often be the need for significant community representation. Consider the case of a system that is governed by a small board that chooses its members based primarily on organizational and governance needs. This system has subordinate boards overseeing organizations that serve local communities. They are composed substantially of individuals from the communities served. Each subsidiary board is charged with the tightly defined responsibilities for credentialing of medical staff, quality of care, and community health and relationships.

In this example, the composition of different boards within the system is based on different principles. The parent board uses the principle of seeking the best, most qualified individuals regardless of where they live or work. The subsidiary boards, with much more constrained responsibilities and roles and local focus, use the principle of community representation as the basis for board composition.

This model provides the opportunity for community representation, but does so at the cost of the disadvantages of decentralized governance. For those systems with a decentralized governance model, this differential approach to board composition can be a workable compromise. It provides a focused parent board composed on the basis of talent and skill, and subordinate boards that are composed first for community representation and second for skill and qualifications.

However, for those systems that are moving toward a centralized or modified centralized governance structure, the differential approach to board composition loses currency. In the modified centralized approach there are fewer subsidiary boards and they have significant governance responsibility. These boards, like the parent, must be composed for maximum governance effectiveness. This again precludes community representation as the primary consideration in board composition.

Pause and Reflect: How Representative Is Your Board?

How many different communities are served by your organization? (Communities may be defined geographically, economically, demographically, or in other ways.) Are each of these communities represented on your board? Of the communities that are represented on your board, why are they there? Of the communities that are not represented on your board, why aren't they? What is the impact of the degree of community representation or lack thereof on your board's performance and contribution?

Clearly, the issue of community representation strikes at the very heart of how health care organization governance is defined. Yet as the industry changes, so too must governance. We believe it is time to examine the deeply held belief that health care organization boards must be composed exclusively—or even primarily—to represent their communities.

Benchmark Practices: Composition

The issue of board composition, at first glance, appears to be a simple, straightforward topic that does not warrant much attention. Nothing could be further from the truth. Just as the rapidly changing

Statement	No	Somewhat	Yes
• New members of my board are selected on the basis of explicit, established criteria.	1	2	3
• The members of my board are limited in the number of consecutive terms they can serve.	1	2	3
• Reappointment to additional terms is based on a member's past performance, board needs, and the organization's circumstances and challenges.	1	2	3
• Member appointment and reappointment decisions are based, in part, on the results of a comprehensive and thorough board profile.	1	2	3
• My board's by-laws or policies prescribe a mechanism and associated criteria for removing a member from office.	1	2	3
• There are no more than two ex-officio members of my board.	1	2	3
• The CEO is a voting member of my board.	1	2	3
• Physician members of my board tend to represent narrow medical interests rather than the organization's stakeholders in general.	3	2	1

(continued on page 184)

Governance Check-Up: Composition

Statement	No	Somewhat	Yes
• My board periodically engages in a formal and thorough assessment of its composition.	1	2	3
• My board is composed of individuals who possess the knowledge, skills, experience, perspectives, and characteristics to effectively govern our organization both now and in the future.	1	2	3
TOTAL =			

Governance Check-Up: Composition
Source: © Orlikoff and Associates, Inc., 1998.

8	10	12	14	16	18	20	22	24

Low
Performance   Moderate
                              Performance   High
                                                            Performance

health care industry requires constant adjustment in organization, it also requires change in the principles and process for composing a board. Members—who they are, why they are chosen, whether they are reappointed to successive terms of office—significantly affect board performance and contributions. Effective boards do not choose their members lightly, they do not renew board members' terms automatically, and they are willing to remove a board member from office for poor performance. Thus effective boards place a greater emphasis on board member selection, evaluation, and term renewal and removal than do their more ineffective—and unfortunately more numerous—cousins. Effective boards develop and use an integrated, continuously improving approach to board composition, which includes basing board member selection and evaluation on the combined use of established criteria and board profiling.

- Clearly define board responsibilities and roles, and make them the foundation for the development of categories of weighted criteria for new member selection.
- Use board profiling to identify areas of need, gaps, and redundancies in member skills and experience. Link the development of the ideal board profile to the resulting selection criteria for new members.
- Performance evaluation criteria for the reappointment of board members to additional terms of office should be developed and used for all board members. Renewal of board member terms should not be automatic.
- Develop a defined process and measurable criteria for the removal of members from office in midterm. Review both the process and the criteria with the entire board annually.
- If your board does not have them, institute and enforce term limits for members. If you have term limits, ensure they are enforced and are periodically reviewed. If local circumstances do not mandate a different choice, use a "3–3" term limit—a three-year term and a maximum of three consecutive terms—for a maximum of nine years of consecutive board membership.
- Clarify the mechanisms for the selection of all members of your board, as well as for the members of all boards in your system. Review this with all boards annually.
- Review the number and type of ex officio members of your board. If your board has more than two, seriously evaluate the reasons for this and attempt to reduce their number. If your system board has ex officio members but the system CEO is not one of them, what is the rationale for this?
- Initiate a full and frank discussion regarding community representation as a basis for the composition of your board. Has community representation been a criterion (either implicit or explicit) for board composition? Why? Are the reasons still valid? Should community representation continue to be a critical criterion for member selection and reappointment?

8

Governance Infrastructure

The systems, processes, and procedures that support a board's work form an infrastructure that is as essential to healthy governance as roads, bridges, and power lines are to the health of the economy. Whatever a board's structure, however it views and discharges its responsibilities and roles, regardless of how it is composed, there are basic elements of infrastructure that must be in place for a board to optimize its performance and contributions.

The Effective Governance Pyramid

The Effective Governance Pyramid (Exhibit 8.1) is a model that any board can employ to enhance its performance and contributions. The base of the pyramid provides the foundation for each successive level of infrastructure, building up to the vision at the apex. The objective of the pyramid is to provide boards the infrastructure they need to achieve their mission and accomplish their organization's vision. The mission is what the organization is. The vision is what the board wishes the organization to become at some point in the future. By framing the Effective Governance Pyramid between the mission and the vision, the board establishes a dynamic, creative tension between the two. It is through this tension that the board creates effective policy, makes meaningful decisions, engages in appropriate oversight, and leads the organization into the future.

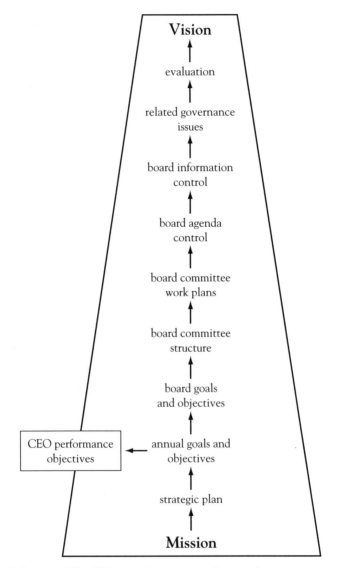

Exhibit 8.1. The Effective Governance Pyramid
Source: © Orlikoff and Associates, Inc., 1996.

The further up the pyramid a board progresses, the more effective it will become.

Mission. Just as the base of any effective health care system is its mission, so too must mission be the foundation of effective governance infrastructure. The mission defines the belief system of a board and forms the foundation for its policy formulation, decision making, and oversight. A good mission helps a board by framing the values, philosophies, and beliefs that define the organization. These serve as touchstones that help a board make consistent and predictable decisions that best support and fulfill the mission.

A fundamental governance responsibility is to develop a meaningful mission and to routinely evaluate it to verify its continued validity. A board must also modify the mission when appropriate, and ensure that the plans and practices of the organization and any subordinate boards are consistent with it.

Strategic plan. A meaningful and clear mission provides the parameters for an organization's strategic plan. Strategic planning is a process of determining how an organization will function consistent with its mission in the face of changing market conditions and other circumstances. It is through oversight of the planning process that a board frames and addresses the dynamic tension between the often conflicting demands of mission and market.

Annual goals and objectives. The strategic plan forms the basis for specific annual organizational goals and objectives. They are benchmarks or targets that, when reached, indicate effective implementation of the strategy. Goals and objectives are tactical and relate to *how* the strategy will be accomplished and measured. The translation of broad strategy into specific, measurable organizational goals and objectives is a keystone of effective governance as it provides focus for both the board and CEO. The goals and objectives are made operational through annual performance objectives.

Performance objectives. A key characteristic of effective governance infrastructure is the clear distinction of the work of the board from that of the CEO. One way this is done is through the development of performance objectives for both. As discussed in Chapter Four, specific and measurable annual CEO performance objectives should be based on annual organizational goals and objectives as well as defined progress toward accomplishment of longer-term strategies. This focuses the CEO's attention and activities on the organization's mission and strategic plan.

Annual Board Goals and Objectives

The first four progressive steps of the Effective Governance Pyramid form the springboard to the next levels, and to the infrastructure of effective governance.

Illustration: Board Goals and Objectives

By the end of this year, our board will:

- Approve a comprehensive plan, with measurable objectives, to improve the health of the communities we serve and devote sufficient organizational resources to begin its implementation.

- Develop and implement a plan to increase board member involvement in key community groups, and to improve community input into our governance process.

- Approve a comprehensive strategy for our future position in the delivery and financing of senior care, receive education and consulting assistance on the advisability of creating a provider-sponsored organization (PSO), and develop a policy on PSO (create, buy, merge, do nothing).

- Develop with the CEO performance objectives and an evaluation process that are more system-focused and less hospital-focused.

- Receive education on the implications of a subsidiary insurance company on the functioning, finances, and governance of our system. Approve or reject a plan for the formation of a subsidiary insurance company.

- Continue our commitment to diversity by expanding the number of women and minorities on our board and its committees.

- Approve a plan for the merger of our two hospital medical staffs into a single medical staff.

Just as the CEO performance objectives focus the CEO's activities, so do the annual board goals and objectives focus the work, time, attention, and structure of the board. The development of objectives for both the CEO and the board clarifies the relative work of each and facilitates an effective partnership.

Boards that do not set yearly goals and objectives for themselves tend to address the same issues and maintain the same structures from year to year, or to focus only on whatever issues or crises that present themselves. Such boards spend most of their time putting out fires and consequently find themselves unable to recognize or effectively deal with patterns of change in the industry and their market.

Explicit board goals and objectives, developed on an annual basis, are the foundation of governance infrastructure. They provide the basis for:

- Constructing board meeting agendas for the coming year

- Determining what will be addressed at board meetings—and what will not

- Creating the board committee structure and charter

- Structuring the information that will flow to the board

- Creating the topical framework and timeline for continuing governance education and retreats

- Fine-tuning criteria for the identification and selection of new board members, as well as for the reappointment of board members whose terms are expiring

- Undertaking board self-evaluation

Board goals and objectives focus board time and attention on action, and on creating the future.

Once the board has developed its annual goals and objectives, it can use them as the basis for determining its committee structure for the coming year. This is done through the zero-based committee design process discussed in Chapter Six. This approach enables a board to tailor its committee structure and functioning to its established, explicit priorities.

Annual Board Work Plans

A key challenge for a board is to strategically align the activities of its committees. Basically, this means that although each committee performs different functions and tasks, the sum total converge to move the board toward the achievement of its annual goals and objectives, and through these, to the organization's achievement of its mission.

To achieve this strategic alignment, a board must do more than simply determine what committees it will have, it must direct its committees. Board committees that lack focus and direction frequently pull the board in many different directions, resulting in governance entropy, which is the opposite of governance alignment.

Illustration: Quality Committee Work Plan

In addition to those activities outlined in the committee description and charge, the board quality committee will by the end of the year:

- Assist management in the development of a comprehensive plan, with measurable objectives, to improve the health of the communities we serve. Recommend a plan for approval to the board.

- Develop an extensive set of community health indicators (at least thirty) including target levels or upper and lower control limits for each indicator, that will be regularly monitored by the committee. Of these, recommend twelve broad indicators of community health for regular review by the board.

- Develop, with the medical executive committees of our two hospitals, a draft unified credentialing process toward the goal of merging the medical staffs next year. Recommend that plan to the board for approval.

- Develop indicators of quality in our outpatient care delivery activities with target levels or upper and lower control limits for each indicator; of these, recommend twelve broad indicators of outpatient quality for regular review by the board.

- Investigate with management the issues and concerns relating to the integration of alternative care providers into our inpatient and outpatient credentialing processes; recommend to the board the advisability of proceeding with this.

A board frames the work of its committees through the use of committee charters (see Appendix B for examples). However, a board fine-tunes committee work through the use of annual committee work plans. The charter or charge describes the functions of a committee, but a work plan explicitly describes its tasks, responsibilities, priorities, and deadlines. Although either the full board or executive committee can develop annual committee work plans, only the full board should approve them. Board goals and objectives are used as the basis for formulating the annual committee work plans. In this way a board specifically controls each of its committees, ensures that their work is facilitating the efficient accomplishment of board goals and objectives, and minimizes wasted time and effort on the part of board members and management. A board might assign several committees different tasks that all relate to accomplishing a specific annual board goal or objective. For example, if a board's objective was to establish a provider-sponsored organization (PSO), it might assign budget development oversight to the finance committee; integrating the PSO into a broader, comprehensive senior strategy to the planning committee; and developing PSO quality indicators and standards to the quality committee. Here, each committee focuses on specific tasks that, when taken together, assist the board in accomplishing its annual goals and objectives.

Board Agenda Control

A board does not really exist unless it is meeting, so the most precious commodity a board has is the time members spend together between raps of the gavel. The art of great governance largely involves maximizing the use of this limited resource. A key way to do this is through control of board meeting agendas.

Pause and Reflect: Your Board's Agenda

Some boards are prisoners of their never-changing agendas. The most mundane, trivial issues come first and take the majority of time. Significant issues, if addressed at all, are placed at the end, when the board members are running out of energy and probably out of time as well.

Try this test. At your next board meeting, take the agenda and cross out the date so that it is unreadable. Have the board secretary bring an agenda from a board meeting two years ago and cross out that date. Now, mix the two agendas up and have the board compare them. Can the board identify the agenda for today's meeting? If the answer is no it implies that the board is addressing the same issues today that it did two years ago—it is a prisoner of its agenda.

An effective board meeting agenda focuses on issues that actually require the board's attention. These issues are identified through the board goals and objectives and work plan. This background planning enables a board to develop a collective sense of what is important, and this is then translated into board agendas for the year. This is why the earlier steps of the Effective Governance Pyramid are such important foundations of board infrastructure: they frame a critical sense of purpose and priority, a perspective of what is important for the organization and for the board. This purpose and priority is then reflected and emphasized in the agendas for board meetings.

A very useful technique involves the use of a *consent agenda*. The board agenda planners (usually the executive or governance committee, but occasionally the board chair with the CEO) divide agenda issues into two groups of items. The first are those items that must be acted on because of legal, regulatory, or other requirements, but are not significant enough to warrant discussion by the full board. Such issues are combined into a single section of the board agenda book; members review these materials prior to the meeting, and if no one has any questions or concerns, the entire block of issues is approved with one board vote and no discussion. This frees up a tremendous amount of time that would otherwise be squandered on minor issues. Any member can request that an item be removed from the consent agenda and discussed by the full board. The success of the consent agenda is predicated upon all board members reading the material in the consent agenda section of the board agenda book. If they do not, then the board becomes a veritable rubber stamp.

The second group of agenda items are those important issues that require discussion, deliberation, and action by the board. These are addressed one by one.

Board Information Control

Effective governance depends upon information that contains appropriate content, is provided in understandable formats, and is tailored to established board priorities. Such governance information is a powerful force in facilitating effective governance. Effective boards control and focus their information; ineffective boards passively respond to whatever information they happen to be given.

Pause and Reflect: Information and Noise

Astronomers categorize data from their radio telescopes and other instruments into two groups: information and noise. The information is studied and acted upon, while the noise is filtered or abandoned. The challenge for a board is to determine what is information and what is noise. We estimate that, on average, about 75 percent of what a health care organization board receives in its agenda materials is noise.

What is the information-to-noise ratio for your board agenda materials?

A governance information system is a cornerstone of effective governance infrastructure. It frames both the content and format of all information provided to a board. The content is framed by the strategy, the organizational goals, and the annual board goals and objectives. The formats are designed to provide information at a level of detail that is appropriate for a board (as opposed to management or clinical information), and that facilitates efficient board review.

There are three broad types of information in health care organizations: managerial, clinical, and governance. Executives need managerial information to run the organization; physicians need clinical information to practice medicine. Likewise, boards need governance information. But what they often get is page after page of mind-numbing (and largely irrelevant) operational detail—by-products of the organization's managerial and clinical information systems, ground out with no thought to the board's specialized requirements. Here are a few of the biggest flaws we encounter:

- Information is not screened and focused to provide the board and its committees with what they really need to discharge their responsibilities and roles, achieve objectives, and accomplish work plans. The information most boards receive is like a shotgun blast, too many pellets flying in all directions with no discernible pattern.

- Information comes to the board in a wide variety of forms and formats; there is little, if any, standardization.

- Full copies of meeting minutes are the primary vehicle committees employ to provide information to the board.

- Data is often presented in column after column of figures rather than portrayed graphically (where trends and variances can be more easily discerned).

- Reports forwarded by management and the medical staff are not preceded by an "executive summary," a succinct description of the recommendation and board action required.

- Far too much information, of the wrong type, is provided.

The last point warrants elaboration. Much of the information a board receives comes from management, the medical staff, and the board's own committees. Say, for example, the board is evaluating the financial health of a fifty-physician primary care group practice that was purchased a year ago. The key features of effective, as contrasted to very ineffective (even dysfunctional), information control are portrayed in Exhibit 8.2.

In an effective system, the CFO might review fifty separate performance indicators, while the CEO examines thirty, the board finance committee looks at fifteen, and the full board periodically monitors only five. By controlling and focusing incoming informa-

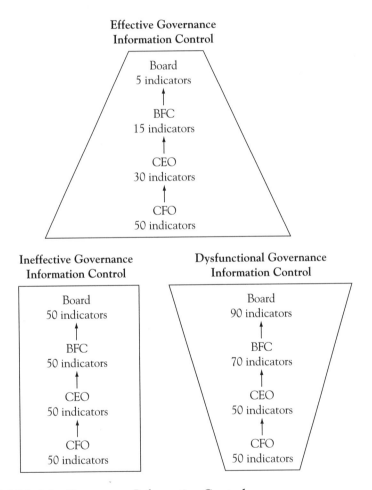

Exhibit 8.2. Governance Information Control
Note: BFC = Board Finance Committee
Source: © Orlikoff and Associates, Inc., 1996.

tion, both the finance committee and the board can exercise appropriate oversight without duplicating (or being overwhelmed by) information monitored and evaluated at lower levels.

Executives and the medical staff have managerial and clinical information systems (MISs and CISs) that provide them the information they require to run the organization—boards must have parallel systems to provide them with the information they need to govern. The specifics of designing and employing a governance information system is a complex topic beyond the scope of this book. If your board lacks this critical element of infrastructure, its design should be included in the board's objectives and work plan. Although the governance literature falls short here, one piece devoted to this topic is the chapter titled "Information and the Effective Board" in Orlikoff and Totten's *The Trustee Handbook for Health Care Governance* (1998). Here are some key points to consider when designing a governance information system.

- The information a board receives should at minimum reflect the current business mix and strategy of the organization. Frequently, the information a board receives relates to how things *were*, not how they currently are or how they will be. For example, it is very common for a hospital to generate, say, 60 percent of its revenues from outpatient care, but have inpatient care information comprise 85 percent of what the board receives. At minimum, the governance information system should ensure that the board receives information that matches the current business mix—and preferably, governance information should lead where the organization is going.
- All information provided to a board should directly relate to and be organized according to the system or organizational strategy and goals, as well as support the achievement of the board's annual goals and objectives.
- Informational reports to the board should be brief and in graphic format whenever possible.

- Board information and agenda packages should be maintained at a reasonable and relatively constant size. If new information is to be added to the package, old information should be deleted. Avoid the common trap of simply piling on more and more information.

- It should be made very clear to a board exactly what the particular information is for. Categorizing information in board agenda books is a very powerful governance information system technique. The following categories are often useful: Monitoring Information, Decision Information, Educational Information, Market Intelligence Information.

- The board should control the content, format, and amount of information it receives. One way to do this is to have the board annually develop and select a series of topic-specific indicators (quality, finance, executive performance, and so on) that it will routinely review. These indicators will allow the board to perform its monitoring functions in a condensed and efficient manner. Once the indicators are selected, threshold or target levels for each of the indicators should be developed. (For example, upper and lower limits can be established for most indicators. If the indicator is within established limits, the board will not spend any of its time reviewing it. If an indicator trend line approaches or exceeds an upper or lower limit, the board will devote attention to it.)

- Indicators, along with upper and lower limits or thresholds, should be presented to the board in graphic format. This facilitates quick board review of the indicators, while providing a big-picture view of the issues.

- An annual calendar for the reporting of routine or required information to the board should be developed and approved by the board at the beginning of every year. Many issues (such as medical staff credentialing, quality reporting, CEO performance evaluation, and regulator-required board reports) that the board must address can be anticipated. These routine reports can then be scheduled for presentation to the board in sequenced and manageable detail through use of an annual board reporting calendar.

- The minutes of meetings of groups other than the board (including board committees) should *never* be a primary vehicle for providing information to a board. (Meeting minutes only have value for the group whose meeting is reflected in the minutes. The only minutes a board should review are those of its own meetings.)
- As part of the annual board self-evaluation, the board should evaluate its governance information system and continually refine and fine-tune it.

Effective boards explicitly control and structure the content, format, and volume of information they receive. They ensure that their information is relevant to the strategy and future of the organization and is in the context of the changing health care environment. The way they do this is through a critical piece of governance infrastructure: a meaningful governance information system.

Evaluation

Evaluation is the activity that integrates and assesses the earlier steps of the Effective Governance Pyramid. Annual board goals and objectives form the basis for the annual board self-evaluation, while the CEO performance objectives form the basis for the CEO performance evaluation.

The interdependent governance-management leadership relationship is framed by establishing related objectives for the board and the CEO at the same time. So, too, should the two evaluation processes be conducted together. Thoughtful CEO performance evaluation and board self-evaluation processes help both the board and management improve their performance and achieve and maintain excellence in governance and management. A board's evaluation of its own performance, structure, and functioning is perhaps the most important infrastructure of effective governance. An honest, well-constructed self-evaluation process, conducted regularly and tied to the implementation of action to improve governance, can help a board achieve and maintain excellence.

Self-evaluation provides a board with the measures both to look back and to plan ahead, answering such questions as What are we doing well? What could we be doing better? To what extent did we achieve our goals and objectives? A board uses the answers to these questions to develop an action plan to improve its performance and establish new goals for the coming year.

Most board self-evaluation processes are based on the use of questionnaires or survey forms anonymously completed by each board member. The aggregate responses are then analyzed and used to facilitate discussion among the board members. A number of issues and concerns typically spring from the facilitated discussion, forming the basis for the development of a governance improvement action plan. Effective action plans outline and prioritize the areas to be strengthened by the board, and set deadlines and responsibility for each action item. The action plan is key to improving the performance of the board, as evaluation without improvement is an empty exercise.

Most board self-evaluations are conducted annually or bi-annually. However, an important aspect of effective evaluation is ongoing governance review. An example of this is the routine post-meeting evaluation conducted by many boards, discussed in the Board Meetings section of this chapter.

When both the board self-evaluation and the CEO performance evaluation are concluded, the annual process of the Effective Governance Pyramid is also complete. The process then begins again for the coming year.

Related Governance Issues

The Effective Governance Pyramid also incorporates many other key elements of infrastructure, including new board member orientation, job descriptions, continuing board education and retreats, and board meetings.

New Board Member Orientation

Effective boards require effective board members. The more quickly a board can bring its new members up to speed the better it can build a cohesive governance team. The best means for doing this is designing and conducting a meaningful new member orientation program.

Orientation is a structured process to develop the knowledge and skills of the new member, and to clarify and instill the cultural norms of the board. It includes content relevant to the unique characteristics of the organization and the board, a clearly defined process for conducting the orientation, and an ongoing evaluation that results in its regular refinement and occasional revision.

Although many orientations are conducted solely by the CEO, the board should oversee and be involved in the process through the executive, governance, or nominations committee. A crucial component of an effective orientation process is to socialize new members to the culture and functioning of the board and thus it is important that board leaders be involved in conducting key aspects of it.

Pause and Reflect: Board Orientation

- How were you oriented to your board?
- How effective was the orientation in preparing you to be a contributing board member as quickly as possible?
- How could the process be improved?

An excellent orientation technique is to have new members attend a board self-evaluation session or retreat scheduled soon after they assume office, sitting in while established members examine board functioning, structure, composition, and infrastructure. This will do more than any amount of reading or briefing sessions to help the newcomers understand the board's view of its own strengths and weaknesses, and become familiar with board values and the relationships among members and between the board and the CEO. The interaction of new members with future colleagues outside the structure of board meetings helps build relationships, rapport, and cohesiveness.

An effective orientation has clearly defined content that provides a foundational understanding of the health care field and is directly related to the mission and strategic direction of the organization, and to the board's own goals and objectives. At minimum, an orientation should address the following:

- A review of the U.S. health care field—its history, financing, and delivery arrangements, and an examination of the recent revolutionary changes in the system. Also included should be a review of national, regional, state, and local health care issues and trends.

- An overview of the organization's market, competitors, and purchaser relationships.

- A review of the communities the organization serves, and its key stakeholders.

- A review of the organization's relationships with physicians and physician groups.

- A review of the organization's vision and mission, key goals and core strategies, and its most significant challenges.

- A detailed review of the board's responsibilities and roles, structure, composition, and infrastructure.

- An examination of the board's culture, key policies, goals and objectives, and work plan.

- A review of the organization's management and clinical structures.

- A review of board member liabilities as well as the protections the organization provides (director and officer insurance, indemnification, and statutory immunity).

Effective orientation is best regarded as a process rather than an event. This process should extend over many months and use a variety of approaches, such as lectures, meetings, videotapes, written materials, retreats, one-to-one discussions, attending the meetings of different board committees, and participation in outside education programs.

The orientation process should be evaluated every few years to verify its effectiveness in preparing new members for their demanding roles. It should be fine-tuned whenever opportunities for improvement emerge.

Job Descriptions

Confusion regarding board responsibilities and roles is a common cause of ineffective governance. This is often compounded by confusion regarding the board's job in relation to that of management and the medical staff. To compound the problem, functions of the board chair are often vague and poorly understood.

For a board to do its job well, its members must share a clear understanding of exactly what that job is. This shared understanding will vary with every board as each has a subtly different scope of authority and definition of its responsibilities and roles, as well as a different mix of skills, personalities, and challenges. To create this shared understanding, each board must answer a basic question: What is the job of the board in *this* organization?

This question is best answered through the creation of a written job description for each board, board member, and board leader. Board job descriptions are a practical part of the infrastructure, assisting in many governance functions from new board member orientation to board self-evaluation. More important, a good job description allows board members to rapidly detect when the board is drifting away from its responsibilities or roles, or is inappropriately treading on management turf. It allows a board to continuously fine-tune its performance by comparing what the board should be doing with what the board is actually doing. A board job description tells potential members precisely what is expected of them should they join the board. Further, the job description tells those who have served on other boards how this board is distinctive. In systems having a decentralized governance structure, job descriptions are invaluable in preventing conflict and gridlock between boards by clearly delineating the relative responsibilities and roles of each.

A meaningful board job description should outline the primary responsibilities of governance, and then specify the roles of the board in discharging them. It should clarify the distinction between governance and management. Finally, it should clarify differences in the responsibilities, roles, and authority of different boards in a system.

Board Chair Job Description

High levels of governance performance and contribution depend on the quality of leadership, yet many boards lack a definition of exactly what the chair is supposed to do. When this is the case the effectiveness of the board fluctuates as a function of changing board chairs.

A precise board chair job description provides one way for a board to hold its chair accountable. The "that's not how I see my job" defense—frequently used by board chairs in delicate situations—cannot be employed in the face of a clear position description. A board chair job description also provides a foundation for orientation and evaluation. Just as new board member orientation and board self-evaluation are critical elements of governance infrastructure, so too is chairperson orientation and performance evaluation. Yet most boards have no such processes simply because they have no job description to orient to or to evaluate performance against.

Illustration: Board Chair Job Description

While general parameters of the position are described in the bylaws, its purpose, responsibilities, qualifications, term, and selection procedures are specified here as board policy.

Purpose

The chairperson, working cooperatively with the CEO, provides leadership to the board; that body ultimately responsible for protecting and advancing the interests of stakeholders. The board chair, along with the CEO, serves as symbol of the organization to both internal and external constituencies. Working closely with the CEO and chief of the medical staff, the board chair is considered to be a member of the organization's most senior leadership team. This is a critical position that has a significant impact on board performance and contributions and, ultimately, on the organization's success.

Responsibilities

Key responsibilities of the board chairperson include, but are not limited to:

- Serving as chair of the board's executive committee (tasks of this committee are described in its charter)

- Serving as chair of the board's executive performance and compensation committee (tasks of this committee are described in its charter)

- With advice and consent of the executive committee, designating chairs of other board committees

- Serving as an ex officio member of all board committees (although, except in the rarest instances, not expected to participate in their work and deliberations)

- Serving as the board's primary representative to key external and internal stakeholder groups

- Serving as a counselor to the CEO on matters of governance and board-executive relations

- With assistance provided by the executive committee:
    specifying annual objectives for the board
    developing the board's work plan
    formulating agendas for all board meetings

- Facilitating board meetings, ensuring that they are focused, creative, effective, and efficient for the performance of governance work

- Serving as a mentor to other board members

- Serving as the board's exclusive contact with the media

- Assuming other responsibilities and performing other tasks as directed by the board

Key Qualifications

- After careful self-assessment and reflection, have the time and energy to assume this demanding position

- Have at least four years of experience as a member of this board

- Possess in-depth knowledge of:
    the health service industry and our local markets
    the organization's structure, functioning, and programs and services
    the governance process

- Have been rated as "outstanding" on the two preceding board member performance evaluations

- Have no overarching conflicts of interest that would prohibit the individual from acting in the best interests of the organization and its stakeholders

- Be respected for personal and professional integrity, wisdom, intelligence, and judgment by the board, management team, and physician leaders

- Have a collegial working relationship with the CEO

Term

The tenure of the board chair shall be a single two-year term. If an individual's term as chair exceeds the maximum board member term limit, that limit shall be extended by the number of years necessary for the individual to complete the term as chair.

Nomination and Election

Nominees for the position of chair need not have served as the board's vice chair or secretary; it is advisable (although not mandatory) that they have served at least one term on the board's executive committee. A special committee shall forward to the board one or more nominees for the position of chair. This committee shall be composed of the present board chair, the CEO, one physician board member (elected by the full board), one at-large board member (elected by the full board), and one past chair, not now sitting on the board (elected by the full board).

Board Member Job Descriptions

Of those organizations that have a job description for the board and the chair, very few have one for members. This is one reason that many boards are composed of members who have very disparate ideas about what they should be doing. A statement of what is expected of each board member—and what is appropriate and inappropriate behavior—goes a long way toward developing a coherent board culture and aligning the members into a cohesive governance team. We strongly recommend that every board take the time to develop a job description for its own members, and to review it periodically to make sure it stays up to date.

Board Retreats

Most health care organizations conduct regular board and leadership retreats. (Some, not liking the military connotation of the term *retreat,* call them *advances.*) Retreats provide a unique opportunity for board education and facilitated discussion, and a focused forum for considering critical issues and achieving consensus outside the structure and time pressure of a board meeting. Regular retreats are a crucial element of infrastructure that helps boards grow, change, and become more effective. There is, however, a big difference between simply conducting a board retreat and designing a successful one.

Successful retreats have specific objectives and are planned to address specific issues. They are designed around the answers to specific questions:

Is the purpose of the retreat . . .

- Primarily educational (and if so, what are the specific learning objectives)?

- To focus on, discuss, and refine board responsibilities and roles?

- To conduct a self-evaluation and develop specific action plans to improve board performance?

- To develop annual board goals and objectives and a work plan?

- To review, debate, and affirm or revise strategy (for example, discussing a potential merger and developing requirements for such a deal)?

A retreat with no specific purpose or objective is following a recipe for failure.

Perspective: Board Retreat Objectives

We are often called in to conduct board retreats. Our first question is: "What do you want us to speak on or facilitate?" A surprising number of clients respond to this by saying: "Oh, whatever you think is important or just do what you usually do at retreats."

It doesn't matter what we think is important. What matters is what the board thinks is important!

What issues or concerns are most pressing? What problems and opportunities must be explored? What new developments and trends need to be better understood? Is it time to conduct a board self-evaluation? Is there conflict that needs to be resolved?

Frequently, a board retreat will suffer from one or more common mistakes in planning or execution:

A lack of clarity in exactly who the retreat is for. If it is to be a *board* retreat, then only board members and the CEO should participate (though spouses can be invited to the social events and meals). If it is to be a *leadership* retreat, participants will typically include the board, physician leadership, and members of the senior management team. Many board retreats are diluted and spoiled by including too many individuals who are not board members.

Holding the retreat in the usual board meeting location. A new, distant environment for a board retreat can create a more relaxed atmosphere, more conducive to free discussion and effective group process.

Attempting to cram too much into the agenda. When too many topics are addressed and an official meeting of the board is planned, the result is a rushed and often frustrating experience.

Having the CEO or other senior executive facilitate the retreat. This precludes the CEO from participating as an equal and may lock the board into the same dynamic that exists during board meetings.

When the CEO, board chair, or other internal person tries to facilitate a board retreat, problems frequently surface as a result of lack of objectivity, perceived or real hidden agendas, or personality conflicts.

Having an agenda that is too rigid. Often, the value of retreats comes from taking the time to explore new issues or address unanticipated concerns expressed by board members in moments of candor absent the time pressure experienced in scheduled board meetings.

Failing to include social and recreational time during the retreat. Time off helps build interpersonal relationships and team spirit that translate into more effective boards. It also allows for informal processing of what was presented and discussed during formal portions of the retreat. Much of the value of board retreats comes from such interaction and relaxed reflection.

Failing to develop an action plan. Even if the primary purpose is educational, effective retreats result in changes in board functioning, structure, composition, and infrastructure. They conclude with agreement on the specifics about what will be changed and done—focused action planning.

Allowing those who did not attend the retreat to derail the action plan. When a retreat action plan is implemented or formally approved at a subsequent board meeting, those members who failed to attend will often ask to be read in to the underlying rationale for the action plan, and may then argue against it. In either case, a board wastes time and risks deflection explaining and defending what was previously decided. The action plan should be briefly explained along with the statement "if you want to have input perhaps you should attend the next retreat."

Perspective: Winning Board Retreats

Collectively we facilitate about sixty board retreats a year. Here are some characteristics of the best:

- Retreats should be carefully planned based on board input; they are not designed *by* management *for* the board.

- Do it with class. Seize the opportunity to use the retreat for expressing appreciation to volunteers who have given generously of their item and energy. Put *everything* on the master bill.

- Invite spouses and significant others.

- Schedule the retreat for two or three days over a weekend at a resort location within easy driving distance of the organization. Mix educational and discussion sessions with time for relaxation. Make sure that all meals are communal to facilitate informal interaction among attendees.

- Don't overpack the days; leave afternoons free or available for recreational activities.

- Don't do things during the retreat that can be easily accomplished back home.

- Include some type of event that celebrates the board's dedication and accomplishments; build team spirit and culture.

- Ensure that every session is superb in terms of both content and style.

- Make all retreat sessions participative. Nothing is worse than passively sitting and listening for several days (no matter how good the speakers).

- If you are planning to use an outside facilitator, make the arrangements far in advance. The best talent book up to 50 percent of their engagements a year in advance. We continue to be amazed when someone calls us and says: "Our retreat is in two weeks, are you available?"

Education of a board and development of its members is not concluded with the orientation process and retreats. Ongoing education is a critical element of governance infrastructure, especially in times of revolutionary change. Thus, regular education programs, external educational events, subscribing to publications and video-tape series designed especially for health care organization board members, and membership in health care governance Web sites are all part of a necessary continuing education process that helps boards improve (see Appendix C for some suggestions).

Board Meetings

As a board only exists when it meets, planning and conducting pro-ductive meetings is a critical element of great governance. One of the key tasks of a chair is facilitating meetings—combining and blending what members do during them so the whole is greater than the sum of the parts. Yet most chairs have not been trained how to do this, and few members know how to evaluate meetings or sug-gest how they can be improved.

Long, rambling, inconclusive, and inefficient meetings are a chronic complaint of many board members. If the chair allows one or two individuals to dominate the discussion or lets the board become sidetracked by incidental issues, meaningful meetings are essentially impossible—and these problems appear amazingly often. Effective, efficient, and creative board meetings are the result of a clear purpose, a focused agenda, summarized governance informa-tion, and an explicit process for formulating policy, making deci-sions, and engaging in oversight.

Here are a few high-leverage recommendations for improving the effectiveness and efficiency of meetings:

- Develop and review specific objectives for each meet-ing. Members often come to meetings with different expectations; clearly stating objectives at the outset creates focus and purpose. Meeting objectives should flow from the board's annual work plan.

- Link the agenda to the meeting objectives. The agenda should make clear distinctions between action, information, and education items.

- Have a timed agenda for each board meeting, and distribute it to all board members prior to the meeting. Efficient meetings are the result of good preparation. Developing a focused, action-oriented agenda is the best way for a board chair to prepare for a meeting.

- Create a realistic agenda that is not packed with too many items. The most important agenda items should be placed at the front of the agenda and accorded the most time.

- Once an agenda is developed, it must be adhered to. Chairs should keep a tight rein on digressions, side discussions, and attempts to bring up issues that have already been addressed or will be addressed later.

- Adhere to meeting start and end times. By firmly sticking to beginning and ending times, the board makes meetings more efficient, and board members are not likely to feel that their valuable time is being wasted.

- Consider holding board meetings in the morning when everyone is fresh, rather than at the conclusion of what for many is a long, grueling work day.

- Never back up and summarize what has gone on in a meeting for someone who has arrived late. This reinforces tardiness and wastes the time of those who were prompt.

- Do not verbally summarize information contained in the agenda packet; assume it has been read and ask members if they have any questions.

- Do not hold meetings concurrently with meals. This all-too-common practice makes it hard to stay on topic, squanders time, and often ruins the digestion!

- Use a clear and defined process to codify policies and decisions.

- Hold board meetings in a room that allows members to see and hear one another without moving or raising their voices.

- Establish that the role of the chair involves attempting to involve all members and to prevent any individual from dominating discussions.

- Conclude each board meeting with a brief evaluation of how the board planned for and used its time. In this process, each board member briefly answers questions that assess the meeting. The results are analyzed by the chair and executive committee to fine-tune future meetings. Meeting evaluation questions could include:

  Did the agenda book contain useful information in the right form that genuinely helped members understand issues? What should be done differently and better in the future?

  Did every board member come to the meeting prepared?

  Did the agenda focus on the organization's vision-driven priorities as reflected in the board's objectives and work plan?

  Did all the members have an opportunity to express their views?

  Did the board spend more time focusing on the future than the past?

Was the meeting challenging and productive?

What specific board member behaviors contributed most to the board's performance and contributions? What behaviors were deleterious?

Did the board chair's leadership of the meeting contribute to its effectiveness and efficiency?

One characteristic of effective decision-making groups is that they decide how decisions will be made. Board meetings are often rendered ineffective when different members have different ideas about the board decision-making process. Effective boards have a clear, agreed-upon process that they routinely use to frame and make decisions. This process addresses such issues as:

- How much discussion is encouraged prior to a vote? Are all members encouraged to speak, or are established positions articulated by designated individuals?

- Which issues, if any, require a supermajority vote? (That is, when is a designated percentage in excess of 51 percent required to carry the issue?)

- Does the board have a policy that, except in emergency or rare situations, it will not vote on issues at the same meeting where the issue is first presented or discussed? (We recommend such a policy.)

Benchmark Practices: Infrastructure

The very best boards have critical systems and processes in place that underpin their functioning, structure, and composition. This infrastructure has been consciously and carefully designed, not allowed to evolve haphazardly. It is grounded on the organization's mission and key goals, and it is directed toward fulfilling the vision.

Statement	No	Somewhat	Yes
• Each year we develop specific board goals and objectives.	1	2	3
• Goals and objectives are translated into annual board and committee work plans.	1	2	3
• My board controls the nature and amount of information it receives.	1	2	3
• My board's meeting agendas are carefully planned and based on our annual objectives and the work plan.	1	2	3
• My board's meetings are creative, effective, and efficient.	1	2	3
• Our chair's leadership enhances the board's performance and contributions.	1	2	3

(continued on page 219)

• Develop and use a structured process, such as the Effective Governance Pyramid, to design, employ, and assess critical elements of infrastructure.

• Put the organization's vision, mission, and key goals on the first page of every agenda book. The second page should list the board's annual goals and objectives. Further, the first several pages of every committee agenda book should contain the committee's charter and work plan. In this way the priorities and purpose of the board and its committees are clear to all and can be employed as a template to focus and organize their work.

• Develop an annual calendar for performing routine functions and reporting required information to the board. Many issues (such as medical staff credentialing, quality assessments, CEO performance evaluations, and regulatory reports) are easily anticipated.

Statement	No	Somewhat	Yes
• New member orientation and board continuing education activities are carefully planned and effective.	1	2	3
• My board engages in periodic and comprehensive evaluations of its performance and contributions that result in the formulation of governance improvement action plans.	1	2	3
TOTAL =			

Governance Check-Up: Infrastructure
Source: © Orlikoff and Associates, Inc., 1998.

| 8 | 10 | 12 | 14 | 16 | 18 | 20 | 22 | 24 |

Low
Performance

Moderate
Performance

High
Performance

These routine functions and reports can then be scheduled for presentation, discussion, and action by the board in a sequenced and manageable manner through the use of an annual board calendar.

• To establish and reinforce the practical distinction between governance and management, and to emphasize the interdependence of the board-CEO relationship, develop the annual CEO performance objectives and the annual board goals and objectives at the same time. Further, both the board self-evaluation and the CEO performance evaluation should be conducted simultaneously.

• Schedule the new board member recruitment and orientation process to coincide with the annual board retreat. New board members should attend the annual retreat within three months of taking their seats.

- Conduct quick evaluations after every board and committee meeting. Collate the results and periodically share the results with members—then engage in some focused action planning to continuously improve meetings. The executive (or governance) committee and board chair should routinely monitor the results of these mini self-evaluations.
- Conduct regular board and leadership retreats. Board retreats should involve only board members and the CEO. Leadership retreats can involve the members of subsidiary boards, as well as physician leaders and senior executives.
- Make board education a line item in the budget. Require that board members meet a minimum continuing governance education requirement to be eligible for term renewal. Offer relevant subscriptions, videos, and Web site memberships to board members to help keep them abreast of health care industry and market trends and governance issues.
- Governance oversight information should be in graphic format whenever possible, and should contain benchmarks, targets, minimums, and maximums to facilitate analysis and interpretation. Narrative reports should always be preceded by a one-page executive summary. The minutes of the meetings of groups other than the board (board committees, medical staff committees, other boards) should never be used as the vehicle for communicating information to a board.
- Develop written job descriptions for the board, the chair, and individual members. These descriptions should be provided to each board member in a policy and procedures book, and should be reviewed annually.

9

Board Membership

Although structure, functioning, composition, and infrastructure are all critical, the quality of governance ultimately depends on what board members do—their practices and behaviors. Board members are the essential resource of governance—they're the only ones who can accomplish board work. Here we address what you can do to become a better board member. We begin with yet another assessment tool and then present some ideas for enhancing your personal performance and contributions.

How Are You Doing?

Complete the following inventory. Of all the ones in the book, this is the most personal. Accordingly, make every effort to be candid and honest in responding to each of the items.

(Text continues on page 229)

Basics

Statement	No	Somewhat	Yes
• I have the time, energy, and level of commitment to be an active and engaged member of this board.	1	2	3
• Over the last year, I have missed more than 20 percent of my board's meetings.	3		1
• Over the last year, I have attended at least 80 percent of the meetings of committees on which I sit.	1		3
• I have no professional or personal conflicts that would seriously jeopardize my ability to act in the best interest of the organization and its stakeholders.	1	2	3
• When a conflict of interest arises, I acknowledge it and then totally remove myself from board deliberations regarding the matter.	1	2	3
• I have talked with outsiders about confidential organizational or board matters.	3	2	1
• I never represent narrow interests or interest groups; my overarching obligation as a member of this board is to serve the organization's stakeholders as a whole.	1	2	3

Subtotal (Basics) = ☐

(continued on page 223)

Context			
Statement	No	Somewhat	Yes
• I understand the major forces and trends affecting the financing and provision of health care services in the United States.	1	2	3
• I understand the basic features of providing and financing health care services through managed care arrangements and the challenges these arrangements pose for the organization.	1	2	3
• I understand the factors that most affect the health status of individuals and populations.	1	2	3
• I understand the demographic, social, and economic characteristics of the organization's markets.	1	2	3
• I understand the characteristics, strengths, and weaknesses of the organization's key competitors.	1	2	3
• I have a thorough understanding of the organization—its structure, major programs, finances, and operation.	1	2	3
Subtotal (Context) =			

(continued on page 224)

Board Membership Check-Up

Preparation

Statement	No	Somewhat	Yes
• I subscribe to—and read—at least one health care–oriented magazine in order to keep abreast of developments in the industry.	1	2	3
• I participate in board education and development activities conducted by the organization.	1	2	3
• Within the last two years, I have attended an extramural governance-focused educational seminar.	1		3
• Within the last year, I have asked the CEO or staff to provide me with background information (articles or reports) on a specific issue I needed to understand better.	1		3
Subtotal (Preparation) =			

Responsibilities

Statement	No	Somewhat	Yes
• I am familiar with the organization's key stakeholders and understand their interests and expectations.	1	2	3
• I understand and am able to support the organization's vision (its core purposes and values).	1	2	3
• I understand the organization's key goals and major strategies.	1	2	3

(continued on page 225)

Statement	No	Somewhat	Yes
• I keep the vision as foreground when participating in board policy formulation and decision making.	1	2	3
• I know the details of our CEO's compensation package (base salary, incentives, benefits, and perks).	1	2	3
• I avoid becoming involved in managerial and operational matters.	1	2	3
• I have confidence in our CEO and top management team.	1	2	3
• I understand the factors that most affect the quality of care provided in the organization.	1	2	3
• I understand the process and criteria employed to appoint, reappoint, and determine the privileges of physicians.	1	2	3
• I am able to read and interpret the organization's financial statements (balance sheet, income and expense statement, cash flow statement).	1	2	3
• I have a general understanding of the organization's budget and the way in which resources are deployed across major programs and activities.	1	2	3
• I have reviewed my board's by-laws in the last two years.	1	2	3
Subtotal (Responsibilities) =			

(continued on page 226)

Board Membership Check-Up

Meetings			
Statement	No	Somewhat	Yes
• I carefully and thoroughly review all background materials prior to board meetings.	1	2	3
• I look forward to attending board and committee meetings.	1	2	3
• I arrive at meetings on time and do not leave early.	1	2	3
• I am alert and attentive during meetings.	1	2	3
• I actively participate in my board's discussions and deliberations.	1	2	3
• I refrain from talking too much and do not dominate discussions.	1	2	3
• I request additional information, ask questions, and seek clarification when I do not understand an issue my board is deliberating.	1	2	3
• I listen to the views of other board members and carefully consider them.	1	2	3
• I ask tough questions when the need arises.	1	2	3
• I am comfortable expressing dissenting opinions.	1	2	3
• When disagreeing with fellow board members, I do so on the basis of the issues—not personalities.	1	2	3
• I vote no when I disagree with a proposed policy or decision.	1	2	3

(continued on page 227)

Statement	No	Somewhat	Yes
• Once my board formulates a policy or makes a decision, I am willing and able to support it regardless of how I voted on the matter.	1	2	3
Subtotal (Meetings) =			

Membership

	No	Somewhat	Yes
• I enjoy being a member of this board.	1	2	3
• I am proud of my board and its contributions.	1	2	3
• My knowledge, skills, and experience are relevant to being a member of this board and contributing to its work.	1	2	3
• Through my membership on this board, I continue to learn new things.	1	2	3
• I familiar with the background, interests, competencies, and values and perspectives of fellow board members.	1	2	3
• I have a collegial working relation-ship with other board members.	1	2	3
• At least yearly, I reflect upon and assess my performance and contri-butions as a member of this board.	1	2	3
• I would be willing and honored to serve an additional term on this board.	1	2	3
Subtotal (Membership) =			

(continued on page 228)

Board Membership Check-Up

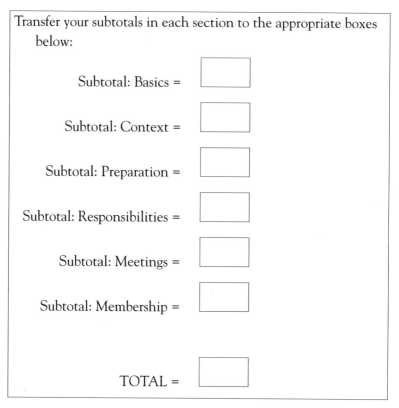

Transfer your subtotals in each section to the appropriate boxes below:

Subtotal: Basics = ☐

Subtotal: Context = ☐

Subtotal: Preparation = ☐

Subtotal: Responsibilities = ☐

Subtotal: Meetings = ☐

Subtotal: Membership = ☐

TOTAL = ☐

Board Membership Check-Up

Source: © Dennis D. Pointer, 1998. Adapted from the Governance Assessment Process (GAP)®. Duplication or use beyond the scope of this book is prohibited.

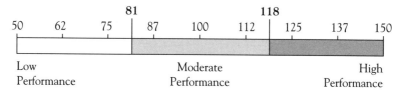

| | | | | | 81 | | | | 118 | | | |
| 50 | 62 | 75 | | 87 | 100 | 112 | | 125 | 137 | 150 |

Low
Performance   Moderate
Performance   High
Performance

Thirty-Eight Really Great Ideas for Becoming a Better Board Member

As we travel around the country giving speeches and conducting board retreats, people constantly ask us how they can become better board members. Almost everybody wonders what specific things they should do—and avoid doing—to make the greatest contribution to their board's work. Here are some of the best ideas we have garnered from our experience as board members and governance consultants:

- Subscribe to *Modern Healthcare* and *Trustee* magazines. These are two of the best sources of industry news, commentary, and governance improvement ideas. Start a clippings file on topics relevant to issues that are important to your board. If you are the CEO or board chair, have the organization purchase subscriptions for each board member; you can find ordering information in Appendix C.
- Attend at least one extramural health care and governance educational seminar every other year. We strongly recommend those sponsored by the American Hospital Association and the Governance and Estes Park institutes; information about their offerings can be found in Appendix C. Many state hospital associations also conduct excellent educational programs for board members.
- If you lack the knowledge to read and interpret financial statements, acquire it immediately. This is one of the most important of the basic competencies that every board member must have. There are a number of great books and self-study manuals available that can help (ask your CEO or chief financial officer for some recommendations). One of the best we have run across is *Finance and Accounting for Nonfinancial Managers*, published by Addison-Wesley; it can be found in most major bookstores.
- Arrange to spend a couple of hours with several representative members of the medical staff and key physician groups. Get a feel for the nature of their professional lives, aspirations, challenges,

perspectives on current health care issues, and assessment of the organization's key strengths and weaknesses.

• Check on the limits and key provisions of your board's directors and officers (D&O) liability insurance coverage, in addition to how you are indemnified (typically described in the by-laws). Be sure to review the "limitations and exclusions of coverage" sections. Ask that your organization's counsel make a presentation on the topic at an upcoming board meeting. The good news: board members of nonprofit health care organizations rarely get sued. The bad news: if you are sued and your D&O coverage and indemnification are not up to snuff, you have problems.

• If you have been recently appointed, expect to serve an apprenticeship before becoming a journeyman board member. You have a lot to learn—about the health care industry, your local market, the organization and the opportunities and problems it faces, your board's culture and the way it works, and governance itself. It takes the most able and committed person with no health care experience at least a year to get up to speed. Be patient. However, remember that you were asked to join this board because you have a contribution to make; when the opportunity arises, do so.

• To quote Martin Luther King, "keep your eyes on the prize." Your overarching and fundamental obligation as a board member is to protect and advance the interest of stakeholders; you are their representative and agent in the organization. Walk in their shoes when you consider issues, policies, and decisions.

• Your board's most important work is discharging its governance responsibilities (for ends, executive management performance, quality, finances, and itself) and roles (policy formulation, decision making, and oversight). Do everything you can to help your board stay on track, avoiding issues and tasks that are irrelevant, inconsequential, or better handled by others. Remember that while tasks and authority can be delegated, governance responsibilities and roles can't.

- Keep your attention focused on the road ahead. To make a difference, you must be future oriented. Become fixated on your organization's vision. Virtually everything you and your board does should be directed toward fulfilling it.

- Remember why you are on the board: to govern the organization, not to manage it. Particularly if you are an executive yourself, it is very easy (and sometimes tempting) to cross the line from directing to operating. Whenever a board slips into management, however, the quality of both governance and management declines.

- The quality of governance can never exceed the quality of information your board receives—constantly assess it in terms of:

Timeliness

Accuracy

Potential bias

What has been left out and unsaid

Unstated assumptions

The frame of reference of whoever compiled it

- Before every board meeting read over and reflect on the vision and key goals. Review the most important issues, recommendations, and proposals that will be discussed during the meeting in light of them. Based on what your board has previously decided matters most (its vision and key goals), ask yourself: What questions should I ask? What should we do and decide to fulfill the vision and achieve our key goals? To really govern, your board's deliberations and actions must be vision and goal driven.

- Come to each board and committee meeting prepared, having carefully read through agenda materials and proposals and recommendations up for discussion and vote. If meeting agenda books do not contain summaries and needed background information, demand they be included in the future. Additionally, you have a right to expect materials forwarded prior to meetings to be carefully prepared, succinct, and sufficient to bring you up to speed before engaging in a discussion and deliberation and casting your vote. Except in emergencies or when matters are trivial, never vote on a proposal you have just seen or heard.

• While participation does not equate to contribution, it is impossible to contribute without participating. Talking is the primary way boards get their work done. Speak up—share your ideas, perspectives, experiences, and values. Encourage others to contribute by asking them questions or seeking their opinions. Board membership is not a spectator sport.

• If you do not understand an issue, always ask for additional information and clarification. Never assume that everyone else is clear about something and you are the only one that isn't. You must fully understand issues brought before the board to fulfill your fiduciary obligation of care (acting as a prudent person would under similar circumstances).

• When dealing with really significant issues, always question and challenge. One of the most important things a board does is to serve as a source of checks and balances when proposals are forwarded to it.

You must be prepared to ask the tough questions. The very best and most helpful questions are those that seek to understand and clarify: which alternatives were considered and discarded (and why); the worst-case scenario if the proposal is implemented; and how the proposal affects and furthers the interests of key organizational stakeholders.

You must be prepared to challenge assumptions. All proposals are based on them, and they are often implicit and fuzzy. Unclear, illogical, or just plain wrong assumptions will sabotage proposals that look wonderful on the surface. Help your board identify and defuse these time bombs.

- Don't be put off by smoke or BS—there is a good bit of both in many boardrooms. Be tenacious in exploring an issue when your gut tells you that all is not right.

- Demand that an adequate amount of board time be spent on the big issues. As Lyndon Johnson once said, "The greatest mistakes generally arise when an important decision passes through a deliberative body like grease through a goose." It is far easier to deal with simple and inconsequential matters; the routine often drives out the nonroutine. When a decision has significant consequences and is risky, demand that the board have the patience to deliberate it properly.

- Always be prepared to express a dissenting opinion and to vote no. Don't be pressured by apparent overwhelming agreement. In light of the facts, after listening carefully to your colleagues and taking a stakeholder perspective, vote your conscience. In the boards on which we have sat, the biggest mistakes have been avoided because one or two members were willing to go against the crowd. If you are the lone dissenter on an important vote, always share your rationale for voting no—and make sure it is accurately summarized in the meeting minutes.

- Don't talk too much. Avoid being the one who dominates every discussion or always says something even when you have nothing meaningful to contribute. The best boards are characterized by relatively even participation across all board members.

- Don't show off; it wastes time and makes you look foolish. Anyone who has sat on a board has seen members asking questions and making comments not to be constructive but rather to demonstrate their knowledge and expertise. Leave your ego at the boardroom door.

- If you are the board chairperson, one of your most important responsibilities is facilitating effective and efficient meetings. Develop the knowledge and skills needed to do this (you're not born with it and most people don't pick it up through experience alone).

Attend a seminar (check with your CEO, state hospital association, or local college) and read a few books on the subject. Several we recommend are: *How to Make Meetings Work* by Michael Doyle and David Straus (Berkley Books); *How to Run a Successful Meeting in Half the Time* by Milo Frank (Pocket Books); *The Strategy of Meetings* by George Kieffer (Warner Books); and *Effective Group Problem Solving* by William Fox (Jossey-Bass).

• Compliment your fellow board members (both publicly and in private) for their ideas, participation, and dedication. It's contagious and builds energy.

• Never ever take action alone, or speak on behalf of the board or the organization unless specifically authorized to do so. Remember, your board exists and can act only as a group. When the game ends, a referee's authority and power evaporates; when a board meeting is over, so does yours. As an individual outside the board-room, don't ever make demands of management, make promises to members of the medical staff or employees, or meddle in operations.

• Do not compromise your ethics and values. A great general principle is: Never do or say anything in the boardroom that you wouldn't want to read about on the front page of your local newspaper the next morning.

• Support your board's policies and decisions even though you do not agree with them, and even if you voted against them. To govern well, your board must speak with a single voice. If you are continually unable to join in the chorus after having sung your song, consider resigning.

• If you have concerns about what your board is doing or how it is going about it, express them. First talk with the board chair. It this does not work, request that the matter appear on the agenda.

• Never perform nongovernance work for your organization, even on an unpaid basis. If you are a real estate professional, you can share your expertise with the board in general terms, but stop short of appraising a building the organization is thinking about purchasing. Likewise, if you are an information consultant, let someone on the staff prepare that RFP for the new computer system, and if you are a journalist, don't spend your time writing a press release about that new program. Doing so, regardless of the contribution you might make, will jeopardize your objectivity as a board member. It will always cause difficulty if your advice is not taken, and—most important—it will blur the line between governance and management.

• Keep your distance from second- and third-line executives, management staff, and employees. Always be friendly, but don't develop any close relationships, personal or professional. The reason: it is essential to scrupulously avoid even the appearance of providing others an opportunity to do an end run around the CEO.

• Be on the alert for instances where your personal and professional interests might conflict (or even appear to conflict) with those of the organization and its stakeholders. One thing is certain: as an engaged and successful member of the community you will have conflicts of interest; they're unavoidable.

Each year, disclose in writing all potentially significant conflicts. Your board should have a reporting form to help you do this.

Acknowledge any significant conflicts as they arise. When a policy or decision is being considered by your board and you have a personal or professional conflict that could prohibit you from acting in the best interest of the organization or its stakeholders, speak up at once. If others (or you yourself) consider the conflict to be material, extricate yourself from all involvement in the matter—leave the room and do not discuss the issue with management or your board colleagues.

• Keep sensitive information that you learn about in your role as a board member strictly confidential; never discuss it with friends, business associates, or family members. If you are uncertain what is confidential, ask. You will rarely get in trouble (or compromise your board and organization) by saying too little.

• When talking to outsiders, remember what your mother always told you: If you don't have something good to say, don't say anything at all. No matter what problems you see with the organization, your board, fellow board members, medical staff, management, or employees, you'll only reduce your ability to help if you air your grievances outside the board.

• Be extremely cautious about how you interact with the competition. Consider appearances—being a regular golfing partner of a competitor's CEO, or being a patient (or allowing a family member to be a patient) in a rival facility will raise questions whether they're justified or not. Pay careful attention to the symbolic aspect of board membership. GM board members don't drive Fords!

• Get to know your fellow board members, including the CEO. Make an effort to understand where they are coming from, the things that are important to them, and what they want to accomplish. Good relationships are powerful elixirs that facilitate how, and how well, a board does its work.

• If you are the CEO or board chair, take each member of the board out to dinner at least once a year. If your board is so large you cannot do this, start working now to reduce its size. A relaxed atmosphere, away from the time pressures of the boardroom, is ideal for getting to know your colleagues, strengthening your interpersonal relationships, better understanding their perspectives and concerns, and talking with them about their performance and contributions.

• Do a personal accounting of your board membership:

What are you giving? Estimate the amount of time you've spent fulfilling your responsibilities during the last year (include everything—traveling to and from the organization, attending board and committee meetings, sitting in on conference calls, preparing for meetings, participating in social events, going to educational programs and retreats, and so on. If you have had any nonreimbursed expenses, total them up.

What are you getting back? Next, construct a succinct list of the benefits that you derive from board membership. Be honest with yourself; consider such things as professional contacts, prestige and recognition, personal learning and development, fellow-ship, a sense of contributing to your community, and so on).

Is there rough parity between your gives and gets? Most of us are quite willing to tolerate a temporary imbalance in costs and benefits. However, when the gap is too big for too long our motivation inevitably declines.

• Once each year, engage in a careful, thoughtful, and critical self-examination of your role as a member of this board. Here are some questions you might ask yourself:

How am I performing? How could I perform better?

How much of a contribution have I made over the last year? What specific things could I do to make a greater contribution?

What are some of the things I do in meetings that impede board performance?

What are some things that I refrain from doing, but shouldn't?

Do I have the time and energy to be an engaged and active member of this board?

Do I still enjoy being a member of this board?

• When you realize that you do not have the time, energy, or commitment to serve on this board, or have had too many instances where you find it difficult (or impossible) to support its policies and decisions—*resign*. Do so gracefully and with style, but do it.

10

Transforming Governance

Based on forty collective years of working with many hundreds of boards, we have come to the following conclusions regarding the governance of health care organizations:

First, boards can make a difference—to the organizations they govern, and to their stakeholders and customers and the communities they serve. Boards bear ultimate responsibility for their health care organizations, and wield ultimate power and authority in them. What they do (or fail to do) and how they go about doing it can have very significant consequences. The operative term here, of course, is *can*. Boards *can* make a difference, but they don't necessarily do so.

Pause and Reflect: Can Boards Make a Difference?

If you have any doubts about our first conclusion, try this thought experiment.

Imagine that at an upcoming meeting, your board is given the following assignment:

You have one hour to formulate policies and make decisions that will really harm stakeholder interests and impair if not destroy the organization. Your objective is to do as much damage as possible in the time allotted. Be creative and totally ruthless in approaching the task. Focus on both the short and long term.

Could your board do it? Of course it could (and it would not take an hour).

Is there any doubt that boards can make a difference?

Second, most boards do not make the difference they should and could. It's not that boards add no value. Rather, they operate far below their capacity and don't make the contributions they are capable of making; talent, energy, and dedication is often wasted. Most board members and CEOs know this, but few admit it and confront the consequences.

Third, the performance and contributions of boards—the difference they make and value they add—can be dramatically enhanced. This requires transformation of, not just incremental improvement in, how health care organizations are governed: different ways of thinking about why boards exist, what they must do, how they should go about it. It requires a fundamental redesign of board functioning, structure, composition, and infrastructure. Boards must reinvent themselves to lead at a time when their industry, their markets, and their organizations are undergoing revolutionary change.

How Does Your Board Rate?

Where your board goes from here, and how it gets there, depends upon its present position. Here is an opportunity to take a navigational fix.

STEP #1. Place numerical scores for the Governance Check-Ups you have completed throughout the book in the appropriate boxes:

Stakeholders (Chapter One, page 10)

Change (Chapter Two, page 20)

Responsibility for Ends (Chapter Four, page 38)

Responsibility for Management Performance
  (Chapter Four, page 52)

Responsibility for Quality (Chapter Four, page 66)

Responsibility for Finances (Chapter Four, page 76)

Policy Formulation Role (Chapter Five, page 94)

Decision-Making Role (Chapter Five, page 98)

Oversight Role (Chapter Five, page 105)

Structure (Chapter Six, page 148)

Composition (Chapter Seven, page 183)

Infrastructure (Chapter Eight, page 218)

STEP #2. Add up the scores from the twelve
check-ups:

Divide the total by 12 and place the resulting average on
the grid:

8	10	12	14	16	18	20	22	24

Low   Moderate   High
Performance   Performance   Performance

The result is an indication of your perception of your board's overall level of performance, and of its need for transformation.

STEP #3. Transfer your scores on the twelve check-ups to the Governance Performance Map (Exhibit 10.1) by placing a dot on each dimension, connecting them as noted in the illustration (Exhibit 10.2).

Governance Performance Map

The map you completed in Exhibit 10.1 is a graphical representation of your board's strength and weakness across those dimensions of governance that have the most impact on its performance and contributions. A truly transformed board—one that really governs,

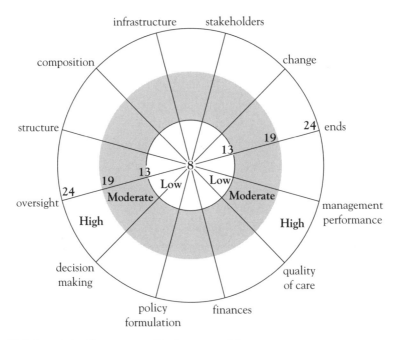

Exhibit 10.1. Governance Performance Map
Source: © Dennis D. Pointer, 1998; adapted from the Governance Assessment Process (GAP)®.

makes a difference, advances the interests of stakeholders, and adds value to its organization—rates in the High zone on each of these twelve dimensions. A transformed board:

- Understands the organization's key stakeholders and their expectations.

- Is able to deal with—and take advantage of—revolutionary changes in the health care industry and its local markets.

- Fulfills its responsibilities for ends, executive management performance, quality, and finances.

- Executes its core roles of policy formulation, decision making, and oversight.

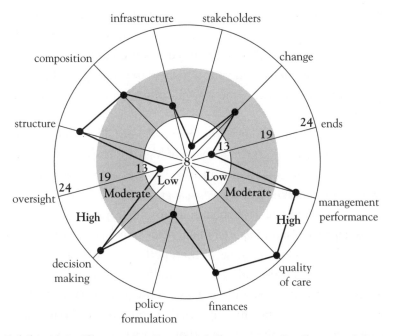

Exhibit 10.2. Illustration: Completed Governance Performance Map
Source: © Dennis D. Pointer, 1998; adapted from the Governance Assessment Process (GAP)®.

- Employs an appropriate governance structure to subdivide and coordinate the performance of board work within the organization.

- Is composed of individuals possessing competencies and capacities that are aligned with organizational challenges and the board's own needs.

- Has the necessary elements of infrastructure in place to support its work.

Based on the ideas and insights you have gained by reading the book, and on your board's plot on the Governance Performance Map, spend some time reflecting on the following questions.

Dimensions on Which You Rated Your Board High

Was your initial assessment candid? Does it accurately portray your board's actual performance and practices? Look over each of the Governance Check-Ups that resulted in a high rating. Review the individual statements and your responses to them. Would you still rate your board in the same way? If not, complete the check-up again.

Would the rest of your board agree with you? The check-ups on which you gave your board a rating of high are based on your individual perceptions and assessments. To what extent do you think your board member colleagues, as a group, would have made the same choices? How might their opinions differ from yours?

What are the most important things that your board must continue doing well? Sometimes areas of high performance do not receive much attention (other wheels are squeaking louder and there's not enough grease to go around) and, as a consequence, gradually deteriorate over time. Has this happened in your board? What specific things should be done to ensure that it does not?

What should your board be doing to celebrate and call attention to those things it does exceedingly well? To build and maintain motivation and spirit, your board must recognize its excellence. Is it doing enough?

Are there any problem areas? Although your overall rating on a given dimension may have been High, there are probably a few check-up items to which you responded "no" or "somewhat." Do not overlook them; these are things your board does not do particularly well that are surrounded and perhaps masked by excellence— a few weeds in a patch of roses. What, specifically, must your board do to correct these problems?

Dimensions on Which You Rated Your Board Moderate or Low

These dimensions (especially those rated in the low range of the scale) deserve your most careful attention. They are features of your board and the way it goes about its work that must be fundamentally redesigned, not just incrementally improved. A transformation must occur if your board is to optimize its performance and contributions, add significant value, and really govern your organization on behalf of its stakeholders. These are your board's greatest developmental opportunities.

Do you think your assessments are shared by your board member colleagues? To what extent might they agree that these characteristics and practices seriously jeopardize your board's performance and contributions? Problems must be recognized before they can be addressed and solved; all significant change begins with a high degree of consensus that change is necessary.

What are the most significant implications and consequences of the items rated low? What is the effect on your board (and other aspects of its performance), the organization as a whole, management, the medical staff and physician partners, and other organizations and boards (if you are part of a system)?

What aspects of governance and practices contributed most to the low rating in each dimension that received one? Carefully review the check-ups for each dimension you rated low. Make a list of them.

What are the most important specific actions that must be undertaken by your board to replace a problematic characteristic or practice with a benchmark one? That is, what are the things your board must do to transform itself? Rough out a series of action plans to address these issues.

Transformation Process

We have helped many boards transform themselves. Although each of these experiences had unique features and challenges, here are some high-leverage recommendations we have found to be widely applicable.

• Realize the process takes eighteen to twenty-four months and will require significant effort. The time and energy expended to mount a transformation must be added to the normal workload of your board and its committees (which cannot be put on hold during the process). Be prepared to work longer and harder for a while—the investment will pay handsome dividends.

• Start by deciding what you need to do. You would not begin remodeling a house without a clear image of what it will look like when it's completed, or without a detailed set of plans—why try to remodel your organization without at least as much thought? Additionally, your board must have a shared understanding of benchmark governance characteristics and practices (an empowering image of what should and could be done) in addition to a map or plan of the types of things that must be done. The most efficient way for your board member colleagues to acquire both is by reading this book. We also highly recommend *The Future of Health Care Governance: Redesigning Boards for a New Era* by Jamie Orlikoff and Mary Totten, and *Boards That Make a Difference* by John Carver (see Appendix C for ordering information).

• The board chair and CEO must be totally committed to, and fully support, the need for transformation if the process is to get off the ground, let alone succeed.

- Hold a retreat to thoroughly deliberate, discuss, and debate your board's performance and contributions and the dimensions of transformed governance: identifying stakeholders and their interests, dealing with change, fulfilling responsibilities (ends, executive management performance, quality of care, finances, and self-management), performing roles (policy formulation, decision making, and oversight), board structure, board composition, and board infrastructure. If you're going to go ahead with confidence of success, the outcome of the retreat should be a recognition by your board of the need for transforming governance, a decision to proceed, and a roughed-out set of objectives and board work plan.

- Select someone outside the organization to help in the process. While a board can incrementally improve its performance on its own, mounting a transformation generally requires the assistance of a highly experienced governance consultant. Throughout this process the board must do the heavy lifting, while the consultant serves as a coach, facilitator, and source of technical expertise. It is important that you select someone who has helped others walk this path.

- Form a board committee to work closely with the consultant and serve as a "center of gravity" for the transformation effort. This committee should have five to seven members including the board chair, chair-elect, and CEO. Keep in mind that the role of this committee is not to act on behalf of the board but rather help the board to act. We recommend that the executive committee not lead this effort, as it has enough to do dealing with the normal flow of governance work. A member of the management team should be assigned to provide staff support to the committee and to work with the consultant.

- Be prepared to conduct a series of full board one-day mini-retreats and work sessions every two or three months throughout the process. Regularly scheduled board meetings are not the best forums for getting the work of transformation accomplished.

- If necessary, focus on redesigning board composition first. The reason is simple. If your board is too large and does not have the right mix of competencies and experience, this—more than any other factor—will inhibit (if not totally sabotage) subsequent steps in the process. Additionally, the success of governance transformation depends on reeducating a board about the nature of governance, the work it must do, and the things it must have in place to fulfill its fiduciary obligations. This is best done with the board that will actually be doing the work rather than one full of people on their way out. Downsizing and recasting a board is one of the most wrenching, difficult, and politically and socially sensitive aspects of transformation. It is also the most disruptive—and therefore best done quickly, before resistance has a chance to harden.

• If the structural model in place involves highly decentralized governance, assess it and if necessary redesign it early in the process—before too much work goes into any of its components. Echoing the content of Chapter Five, we strongly recommend reducing governance layers and the number of boards, moving toward a centralized or modified-centralized structure (depending on the system's maturity and degree of integration).

• If your organization is a health care system with multiple governance entities, focus first on the parent board—its composition, functioning, and infrastructure—before working on any of the others. The parent board is simultaneously a primary focus of the transformation effort and a facilitator of change within the organization's governance system.

• Early in the process, focus on infrastructure; the most important elements of which are board objectives and work plans. Excluding the transformation effort, what are the most critical things your board must attend to over the coming year? What are your plans for accomplishing them?

• Assess and, if necessary, reconfigure the structure and functioning of your board's committees. We suggest that one possible way to begin is by forming committees that mirror your board's ultimate responsibilities: an executive and governance committee, an ends committee (working on vision and goals), a finance committee, an executive management performance committee, and a quality enhancement committee; it is the functions performed, not the names, that are important. Employ a zero-based design process, considering your organization's needs in addition to challenges faced by your board, to form other committees—one of which would be governance transformation. Draft committee charters, objectives, and work plans.

• Your board should try its hand at drafting its charter (see the sample at the end of Chapter Five). In doing so, your board will have to confront and resolve some of the most important and fundamental issues of governance—why your board exists (obligations), what it must do (responsibilities), and how it should go about doing these things (roles). Remember the perils of perfection. The objective is not to produce a perfect board charter, just an adequate one that can be refined over time.

• Board policymaking is the fulcrum of effective governance. Your board must see itself as a policy formulating body; it begins to really govern by employing policy as the primary mechanism for conveying its expectations on behalf of stakeholders. Hold a one-day mini-retreat and work session focused exclusively on your board's policy formulation role. Review, discuss, and deliberate the nature of this role and what specific things your board must do to perform it better. During this session, practice formulating policy by focusing on what are likely to be the easiest policies to draft—those dealing with your board's responsibility for itself. Turn next to a few core policies focusing on your board's most critical expectations regarding executive management performance, finances, and quality. Do not attempt to formulate every policy in each of these areas, just the most important ones. The idea is to develop a base from which to make policy formulation the focal point of your board's work in the future.

• Once you have key policies in place, begin developing a comprehensive set of dashboards—indicators that gauge your organization's performance in key areas—to assist your board in executing its oversight role. Again, your goal here does not involve preparing a fully polished and complete oversight package. We recommend starting out by formulating less than a dozen key indicators and associated standards for each of your board's responsibilities (ends, executive management performance, quality, finances, and self-management). What are the most critical things your board must monitor and assess to ensure that things are working out as expected and promises are being fulfilled?

• Systems employing decentralized or modified decentralized structural models must begin to grapple with how governance responsibilities and roles should be subdivided and shared among the parent and subsidiary boards. As we have noted, structure merely provides a set of containers in which board work is done. Structure provides the context for function and facilitates or impairs it; structure per se does not determine what functions should be performed by which governing entity. Exhibit 10.3 provides a model (based on one introduced in Chapter Five) that lays out the problem of allocating the work of the board.

For each of the board's five responsibilities, and with respect to each of its three roles, the organization must make choices regarding the reserved powers and authority of the parent board and the responsibilities and roles that will be either shared with or delegated to subsidiary boards. What should the parent board be doing? What should subsidiary boards be doing? How should the functioning of parent and subsidiary boards be articulated and coordinated so no important governance work is left undone and so overlaps and conflicts in responsibility, roles, and authority are avoided as far as possible?

For example, with respect to the responsibility for quality, a parent board might choose to retain authority for defining quality (both systemwide and in individual provider organizations), delegate authority for making credentialing decisions to hospital boards, and share responsibility for overseeing the quality of care (where the

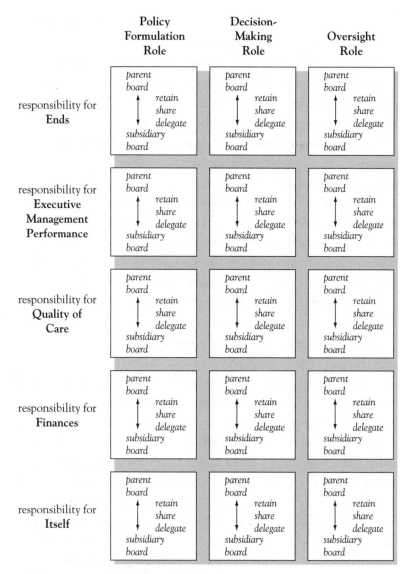

Exhibit 10.3. Subdividing Board Work

Source: © Dennis D. Pointer, 1998; adapted from Pointer and Ewell, 1994.

parent specifies indicators and subsidiary boards employ such indicators to monitor and assess quality).

With respect to the responsibility for self-management, a parent board might choose to retain authority for determining the system's governance structure and setting the size of subsidiary boards, share authority for the composition of boards in subsidiary organizations (where a subsidiary board submits nominations to the parent for approval), or totally delegate authority for determining infrastructure to the subsidiary board.

With respect to the responsibility for management, a parent board might choose to retain authority for formulating policy, making decisions, and overseeing the system CEO; and neither retain, share, or delegate decisions regarding subsidiary organization CEO expectations, performance assessment, and compensation determination. (Since these individuals are direct reports of the system's CEO, these tasks are delegated to him or her.)

This is a complex and time-consuming process, which explains why the vast majority of health care system boards never undertake it. Governance effectiveness and efficiency within systems that employ decentralized structures depends upon a precise and specific mapping of responsibilities and roles among boards. If this is not done, the probability of confusion and conflict increases dramatically. We suggest the parent board (with input from subsidiary boards) craft a series of policy statements specifying how the most important aspects of governance work will be subdivided and shared. These statements need not be perfect, as they can be elaborated and refined over time—but virtually any attempt is preferable to operating on unspoken assumptions until trouble breaks out.

Illustration of Policy Statements: Subdivision of Board Work

- Authority for making credentialing decisions (appointment, reappointment, and delineation of clinical privileges) is delegated to the boards of subsidiary delivery organizations. Subsidiary board quality committees are required to employ system-developed process guidelines and credentialing criteria when they conduct their appraisals and formulate their recommendations. (In an actual policy statement, a specific policy would be cited by number here.)

- Annual subsidiary organization financial objectives, and associated indicators and standards, are developed by system management (in consultation with the subsidiary's CEO and CFO) and reviewed and approved by the parent board. Subsidiary boards are delegated the responsibility of monitoring and reviewing indicators and the extent to which financial objectives are being achieved.

- Subsidiary boards are delegated the responsibility of formulating annual CEO personal performance objectives and assessing the extent to which they have been accomplished. At the conclusion of the fiscal year, the subsidiary board's assessment is to be forwarded to the system's CEO.

- The parent board retains the right to disband and reconstitute (in whole or part) subsidiary boards at any time, for any reason. Members of subsidiary boards serve at the pleasure of the parent board.

The Last Word

Faced with revolutionary change unlike anything experienced since the mid-1960s, American health care is in the midst of a process that will define the future of its own soul: rewriting the values and vision that underpin how health services will be financed and provided well into the next century. This is a time of tremendous challenge and great opportunity. The viability, relevance, and responsiveness of an essential economic and social sector is at stake. Such changes will dramatically shape and be simultaneously shaped by how—and how well—health care organizations are governed.

Continuing to govern large and exceedingly complex health care organizations operating in highly competitive and very unforgiving markets in ways that were developed in a more leisurely past is much like attempting to drive an oxcart on a freeway. A board's ability to influence—and even cope with—profound change in the future depends on its commitment and ability to transform itself—minor alterations and adjustments will not suffice.

In this book we have laid out the key elements of a process that has the potential to transform boards of health care organizations: their functioning, structure, composition, and infrastructure—and, in turn, their performance and contributions.

Governance does make a difference! There is a positive, systematic, and ongoing association between the quality of governance and organizational success. A board can add tremendous value—on behalf of its stakeholders and to its organization. A board can rob its organization of its potential. Which type of board will yours be?

Appendix A
Illustrative Board Policies

This appendix provides a framework for the policy issues a board needs to consider. Each organization's circumstances will be unique, however, and no generic list can cover everything any board might encounter. Thus the material presented here should be regarded as a jumping-off point, not a form to be filled in to create an instant policy package. In addition to defining the specific areas to be covered—which may well differ from the sample text given here—and the individual policies to be applied, the final document would replace the word *organization* with *system* or *hospital,* or the actual name of the institution.

Ends

• The overarching obligation of our board is to represent and serve as agents of our stakeholders by ensuring the organization's resources are deployed in ways that protect and advance their interests. Although the organization has many stakeholders, key ones to which we owe a special fiduciary responsibility are:

• _____

• _____

- _____
- _____

Our vision is an image of what the organization should and could become, at its very best. It has two components: core purposes—the most important things we want to achieve; and core values—the most important principles that guide our decisions and actions.

These are our *core purposes*:

- _____
- _____
- _____
- _____

These are our *core values*:

- _____
- _____
- _____
- _____

- These are the *key goals* the organization must accomplish to fulfill its vision:

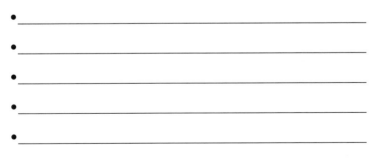

- _____
- _____
- _____
- _____
- _____

Management is accountable to the board for accomplishing these goals.

• Strategies are means employed to accomplish key goals and fulfill the vision. The task of devising strategy is delegated to management. At least two months prior to the beginning of each fiscal year, management is directed to submit its core strategies to the board (via its planning committee). Each strategy must be explicitly linked to one or more key goals and the vision (indicating how it is related to achieving core purposes while simultaneously respecting core values). The board then assesses the degree of alignment between management proposed strategies and the goals and vision.

Executive Management Performance

By end of the fiscal year, the CEO is expected to achieve the following personal performance objectives:

• _____

• _____

• _____

• _____

• _____

• The board's objective is to design a CEO *base compensation* package (excluding bonus) that:

  • Is at the 65th percentile of CEOs in our standardized peer group as determined by the yearly survey conducted by [name of association conducting survey].

  • Is reasonable in light of the organization's circumstances, and is perceived as such by key stakeholders.

- Is motivational, in that compensation (in addition to other factors) influences continuous improvement in performance.

- Rewards the CEO for personal efforts related to achieving performance expectations, accomplishing key goals, and fulfilling the vision (rewards for demonstrated accomplishments in such areas are covered in the board's policy regarding bonus compensation).

- Increases the probability of CEO retention.

- Complies with all applicable laws, regulations, and rulings regarding the determination of executive compensation in nonprofit organizations.

- The CEO's bonus compensation will be drawn from a pool of funds authorized by the board at the beginning of each fiscal year. The dollar amount awarded will be based upon the extent to which baseline expectations have been *exceeded* (as determined by the board's compensation committee), apportioned as follows:

  - Personal performance objectives (weighted by relative importance)—35 percent.

  - Key organizational goals (weighted by relative importance)—65 percent.

- The CEO is prohibited from engaging in, or allowing employees or agents of the organization to engage in, any act that would be judged by a reasonable person to be unethical, imprudent, or illegal, or that violates board policies and decisions.
- The CEO is prohibited from hiring or discharging any executive (at the level of senior vice president or above) without first informing the board. This policy is meant to ensure proper notification of the board, not to restrict the CEO's authority to hire or fire employees.

- The CEO is prohibited from authorizing, without prior board approval:

  - Individual capital expenditures exceeding $XXX,XXX.

  - Expenditures for improvement in facilities exceeding $XXX,XXX.

  - Leases exceeding $XX,XXX in value.

  - Expenditures for new programs exceeding $XXX,XXX.

  - Expenditures for programmatic improvements or enhancements exceeding $XXX,XXX.

  - Contracts for the receipt of services exceeding $XXX,XXX.

  - Contracts for the provision of care services exceeding $XXX,XXX.

The CEO is responsible for formulating prudent authorization limits (less than those noted herein) for other managers and employees.

Quality

- Our board is responsible for ensuring the quality of care provided in and by the organization. We define quality as:

_____
_____
_____
_____
_____

- Based on our definition of quality, at least quarterly, the board (with the assistance of its committee on quality) will monitor and assess the following:

Process and Outcome Quality Indicators

- _____

- _____

- _____

Customer and Purchaser Satisfaction Indicators

- _____

- _____

- _____

Resource Utilization Indicators

- _____

- _____

- _____

Employee and Physician Satisfaction Indicators

- _____

- _____

- _____

Population Health and Disease Indicators

- _____

- _____

- _____

If board monitoring and assessment of these indicators identifies problems, management or the medical staff will be directed to devise and implement a plan to correct them. Such plans must be submitted to and discussed with the board's quality committee.

• All physician members of the medical staff are required to obtain and maintain professional liability insurance in the following amounts:

- • [designated specialty]: $X,XXX,XXX per occurrence and $X,XXX,XXX annual aggregate

- • [designated specialty]: $X,XXX,XXX per occurrence and $X,XXX,XXX annual aggregate

- • [designated specialty]: $X,XXX,XXX per occurrence and $X,XXX,XXX annual aggregate

Such insurance must be obtained from a carrier acceptable to the hospital. Policy provisions must be reviewed by and be acceptable to the hospital's attorney. Each physician shall provide evidence of insurance coverage and premium payment on the policy's anniversary date, when reapplying for staff privileges or when requested. Members of the medical staff are required to immediately notify the hospital of cancellation or changes in coverage.

Finances

• The organization is expected to achieve the following financial objectives in the time frames indicated:

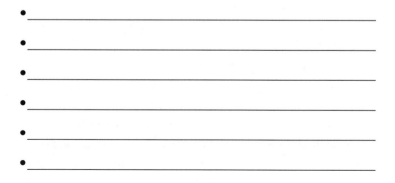

The CEO is accountable to the board for ensuring that such objectives are achieved.

• The CEO is directed to design and implement, by no later than [date], a corporate compliance program to ensure that violations of applicable law and regulations by the organization's employees and agents are prevented or detected and reported. A competent and experienced consultant is to be retained to conduct an annual audit of the program and report to the board regarding the extent to which the organization is complying with its ethical and legal obligations. The report should outline any changes in the program that may be needed to increase its effectiveness.

• At the conclusion of each quarter, the board (with the assistance of its committee on finances) will conduct a thorough assessment of the organization's financial performance employing the following indicators:

Variances (revenue/expense and cash flow statements):

• _____

• _____

• _____

• _____

Financial Ratios (liquidity, activity, capital structure, profitability):

• _____

• _____

• _____

• _____

If board monitoring and assessment of these indicators identifies problems, management will be directed to devise and implement a plan to correct them. Such plans must be submitted to and discussed with the board's finance committee.

- The certified public accounting firm conducting the audit is prohibited from undertaking any consulting engagements for the organization or its subsidiaries.

Self-Management (Governance Effectiveness and Efficiency)

- Policies of the board regarding its own functioning, structure, composition, and infrastructure can be found in the by-laws. The by-laws supersede all policies formulated by the board regarding its own activities.
- Members of the board appointed ex officio (by virtue of a managerial or medical staff position they hold) have the same agency and fiduciary obligations as outside directors: to represent the interest of the organization's stakeholders as a general class. That is, ex officio members are appointed to the board (by virtue of the position held) because they bring expertise and perspectives deemed to be valuable. They are not appointed to represent the special interests of a particular stakeholder.
- Each board member shall exercise good faith and best efforts in the performance of his or her duties. In the performance of duties on behalf of the organization, each director will be held to a strict rule of honesty and fair dealing; no director shall use board membership, or knowledge gained therefrom, in a manner that would create a conflict of interest or the appearance of such. In all matters affecting the organization, each director shall act exclusively on behalf of its interests and shall not knowingly take any position that would adversely affect it. No director shall accept any material compensation, gift, or other favor that could influence, or appear to influence, his or her actions. Each director (by completing the board's annual conflict of interest questionnaire) shall disclose any employment, activity, investment, or other interest that might compete or conflict, or appear to compete or conflict, with the interest of the organization. Each director shall immediately disclose to the board chairperson additional potential conflicts when they arise.

No director shall participate in any discussion, deliberation, or vote where they have a conflict of interest. No director shall, in his or her capacity as a director, claim the status of an agent of the organization unless specifically authorized to do so by the board.

- At least every four years, the services of a qualified governance consultant shall be retained to conduct a thorough audit of the board's functioning, structure, composition, and infrastructure. The consultant shall present recommendations designed to improve the board's contribution and performance.

Appendix B
Illustrative Committee Charters

Committees exist to enhance the effectiveness and efficiency of the board when it meets. Committees cannot assume responsibilities that belong to the board alone. They can, however, help the board fulfill its responsibilities and execute its roles. They do this by performing governance staff work. It is up to the board to ensure that committees function properly. A board does this, in part, by developing charters for each of its committees. This appendix presents some generic illustrations; in practice, the word *organization* would be replaced by *system* or *hospital* or the actual name of the institution.

Executive Committee

The functions of this committee include:

- Taking action in emergency situations where it is not possible to convene a quorum of the board.

- Drafting and forwarding policy recommendations regarding the board's responsibility for ensuring high levels of executive management performance.

- Directing the CEO appraisal process, including establishing annual CEO performance objectives, assessing

CEO performance against these objectives, recommending CEO employment termination if the need arises, and recommending retention of the CEO and adjustment of the CEO's compensation package consistent with the results of the annual evaluation. The executive committee undertakes these activities and makes recommendations to the board for action.

- Developing meeting agendas consistent with the board's annual goals, objectives, and work plans.

Community Health Committee

This committee assists the board in assessing and improving the health of communities served. Its functions include:

- Drafting and forwarding policy recommendations to the board regarding the enhancement of community health.

- Reviewing recommendations management and the medical staff have forwarded to the board dealing with enhancing the health status of communities served.

- Analyzing community health assessment plans and activities of the organization.

- Analyzing plans to improve the health of the various communities served by the organization and presenting them to the board for review and action.

- Developing relationships with community-based groups to integrate activities with them and to establish two-way communication between the organization and the communities it serves.

- Identifying potential collaborative relationships with other community health providers to enhance health status.

- Reviewing community health and morbidity data and making recommendations to the board to ensure that services and resources are aligned with community needs.

- Tracking community demographic, economic, and social trends; identifying implications for changing health care needs; and forwarding these analyses to the board planning committee or the board for integration into the strategic planning process.

Finance Committee

This committee assists the board in maintaining and improving the financial integrity of the system and its subsidiaries. Its functions include:

- Drafting and forwarding policy recommendations regarding the board's responsibility for ensuring the organization's financial health.

- Reviewing recommendations management has forwarded to the board dealing with finances.

- Reviewing the long-range financial plan for the organization.

- Assessing whether the budget is likely to achieve board-formulated financial objectives, key goals, and the vision. Forwarding a recommendation to the board regarding approval, rejection, or revision of the budget.

- Monitoring parent and subsidiary organization financial performance against the approved budget; keeping the board informed of the organization's financial status.

- Developing and recommending a series of financial performance indicators and associated standards for regular review by the board.

- Monitoring financial indicators and presenting analyses to the board when such indicators cross established thresholds or otherwise warrant attention and action.

- Arranging for the annual financial audit by an independent accounting firm.

- Analyzing and presenting to the board major capital plans for the organization and its subsidiaries.

- Recommending corrective action to the board when necessary to ensure compliance with the budget and other financial plans.

Governance Committee

Many boards find it useful to assign the tasks of implementing elements of the Effective Governance Pyramid, presented in Chapter Eight, to a board committee, as opposed to delegating such tasks to different committees. The governance committee assists the board in fulfilling its ultimate responsibility for ensuring its own effective and efficient performance. Its functions include:

- Drafting and forwarding policy recommendations regarding the board's responsibility for its effective and efficient functioning.

- Preparing an initial draft of board goals and objectives.

- Making proposals to the board regarding its committee structure and annual work plans.

- Planning board education, including new member orientation and retreats.

- Developing actual and ideal board composition profiles.

- Identifying potential new board members and making recommendations for their selection to fill vacant board seats.

- Evaluating member performance and forwarding recommendations to the board regarding term renewal.

- Nominating board officers.

- Arranging for, overseeing, and analyzing the results of the governance assessment process.

Planning Committee

This committee assists the board in determining the future directions that the organization and its subsidiaries will take in order to fulfill the vision. Key functions include:

- Drafting and forwarding policy recommendations regarding the board's responsibility for ends.

- Reviewing recommendations from management forwarded to the board dealing with strategies, goals, and the vision.

- Reviewing the strategic plan, making recommendations to the board regarding the extent to which the plan is aligned with board-formulated key goals and the

vision, and presenting the strategic plan to the board
for review and approval, revision, or rejection.

- Ensuring the strategic plan reflects the needs and concerns of subsidiaries.

- Monitoring implementation of the board-approved
strategic plan, and assessing the degree to which the
system achieves its key goals.

- Monitoring parent and subsidiary organization programs and initiatives to ensure consistency with strategies, key goals, and the vision.

- Ensuring that community health needs are addressed in
the planning process.

- Recommending corrective action to the board when
necessary to ensure alignment with board-formulated
key goals and the vision.

Quality Committee

This committee assists the board in overseeing and constantly
improving the quality of care provided throughout the system. Its
functions include:

- Drafting and forwarding policy recommendations
regarding the board's responsibility for ensuring the
quality of care.

- Reviewing recommendations management and the
medical staff have forwarded to the board dealing with
the quality of care.

- Assessing the quality improvement plan for the parent
organization and all subsidiaries, and submitting the
plan to the board for review and approval, revision, or
rejection.

- Assessing the organization's plan to enhance the health of communities served, and submitting the plan to the board for review, approval, revision, or rejection.

- Monitoring quality improvement and community health enhancement plans to ensure fulfillment of the organization's vision-based commitment to quality and community health. Recommending corrective action when necessary.

- Developing and recommending a series of quality and community health indicators and associated standards for regular review by the board.

- Developing and regularly monitoring quality and community health indicators, analyzing trends in such indicators, and recommending corrective action when they cross established thresholds.

- Receiving recommendations regarding applications for appointment and reappointment to the medical staff and delineation of medical staff members' privileges from the medical executive committee of hospitals within the organization. The committee shall compare the recommendations to established criteria for medical staff membership, membership renewal, and privilege delineation. The committee shall then separate recommendations of the medical staff into two groups: (1) those where the recommendations are consistent with the criteria; and (2) those where the recommendations are inconsistent with the criteria or where insufficient information exists to determine consistency of the recommendation with the criteria. The committee shall forward all medical staff recommendations from Group 1 (recommendations consistent with criteria) to the board for action. The committee shall refer all recommendations from Group 2 (recommendations inconsistent with criteria or with insufficient information) back to the medical executive committee, highlighting the discrepancies or areas of insufficient information and requesting that the medical executive committee review and revise the recommendations to make them consistent and complete before resubmitting them to the committee.

- The committee will report to the board summary information and conclusions resulting from its monitoring activities as well as recommendations for board action to improve the quality of care, increase the effectiveness of and quality improvement activities, improve the health of communities served, and minimize the risks of injury to patients and of malpractice losses to the organization.

Appendix C
Governance Resources

The health care field is changing so rapidly that no one can keep up with it from personal experience alone. This appendix lists periodicals, seminars, and books that readers will find useful.

The Best Periodicals

- *Trustee:* The only monthly magazine for health care organization board members. It is published by the American Hospital Association. Subscriptions are $30 per year; call 800–621–6902.

- *The Board Report:* Distributed monthly by Ernst & Young, LLP. Coverage of legislation, regulation, trends and developments, and issues in the industry of interest to health system and hospital board members. Subscription is free; call 800–726–7339.

- *Modern Healthcare:* A weekly health care business news magazine published by Crain Communication. Although targeted at health care management professionals, this is a great source that can help board members keep up with industry developments, trends, and issues. Subscriptions are $125 per year; call 800–678–9595.

- *Healthcare Forum Journal:* Published bi-monthly by the Healthcare Forum, the magazine provides in-depth coverage of various health care issues and organizational innovations. It is one of the best-written publications in the field. Subscriptions are $55 per year; call 415–356–4368.

The Best Seminars

- *The Governance Institute:* 737 Pearl Street, Suite 201; La Jolla, CA 92037 (call 619–551–0144).

  The Governance Institute runs a three and one-half day trustee, physician, and executive leadership conference, held six times each year in various locations across the country. The conferences provide participants an opportunity to exchange ideas with fellow participants, gain new perspectives on leadership roles, better understand emerging issues and industry and market forces, and be exposed to best practices in health systems and hospitals throughout the country. Special sessions are conducted for Catholic organization trustees, spouses, and new board members. The tuition is $950 per participant. Hotel and travel discounts are available.

- *The Estes Park Institute:* P.O. Box 400; Englewood, CO 80151 (call 800–223–4430 or 303–761–7709; fax: 303–789–3896).

  The Estes Park Institute runs a four-day conference for medical staff leaders, executives, and board members, held in various resort locations throughout the country six times each year. Large and small (interactive) groups sessions are led by a distinguished faculty. Follow-up reading materials and videotapes are periodically sent to participants after the program. Registration fee is $1,295; each paid registration includes one free tuition for a community member not directly affiliated with the health care organization. Travel discounts are available with early registration.

The Best Membership Organizations

- *The Governance Institute:* 737 Pearl Street, Suite 201; La Jolla, CA 92037 (call 619–551–0144).

  An education and development subscription service designed exclusively for health system and hospital boards; the cost is $9,500 per year. Benefits include waived tuition for three board members to attend any Institute leadership program (described in "The Best Governance Seminars"); on-demand research services and access to the Institute's governance information clearinghouse; copies of research reports and white papers (the annual surveys of health system and hospital boards); copies of the bimonthly *Board Room Press* for all directors; an annual board self-assessment service that fulfills the criteria of the Joint Commission on the Accreditation of Healthcare Organizations; educational videos on key health care issues, distributed quarterly; a directory of health care speakers who can be employed to plan retreats and educational programs; policy and procedure guidelines; copies of books on governance and health care leadership issues; and tuition-free enrollment at the Institute's annual Chairman and CEO Conference.

- *Volunteer Trustees of Not-For-Profit Hospitals:* 818 18th Street, N.W., Suite 600; Washington, DC 20006 (call 202–659–0338).

A national organization of trustees of leading health systems and hospitals; the only forum run by board members for exchange, discussion, and education. It seeks to help trustees understand the political and economic environment in which their organizations operate and provide them with the tools and information necessary to be effective spokespersons. Volunteer Trustees is a registered lobby committed to preserving and furthering the nonprofit sector of the health care industry and providing a platform from which members can influence public policy. The national trustees' conference, government relations seminars, and committees offer multiple opportunities for exchange. Members receive the *Trustee Newsletter*, specific issue updates, advance notice of upcoming activities, and discounted conference rates. Membership dues are $5,000 per year for health systems or large hospitals, and $2,000 for hospitals under one hundred beds; $1,000 additional for each institution board within a system. Affiliate membership is $500 per year; associate membership is $100.

- *National Center for Nonprofit Boards:* 2000 L Street, N.W.; Washington, DC 20036 (call 202–452–6262).

  The Center distributes a wide variety of books, audio and videotapes, and educational materials; conducts workshops and a yearly National Leadership Forum for board members; publishes the monthly newsletter, *Board Member;* and operates the National Board Information Center (available for referrals, information, and advice). Personal membership is $58 per year; five members of the same board can join for $225 per year.

- *The National Association of Corporate Directors:* 1707 L Street, N.W., Suite 560; Washington, DC 20036 (call 202–775–0509).

  A nonprofit organization assisting those serving on, or working with, boards. NACD is focused primarily on commercial corporations (many of its members are directors and CEOs of Fortune 500 companies), but most of its services are useful to health system and hospital boards. Membership includes subscription to the *Director's Monthly* newsletter; discounts on books, monographs, surveys, and reports; an opportunity to attend the annual NACD Corporate Governance Review program; discounts on more than thirty education programs offered throughout the country each year; the *NACD Director's Register,* a listing of board openings and individuals presently serving as directors; and access to the Corporate Governance Advisory Service, which offers assessment and consulting services. Individual membership is $425 per year; a board can join for $375 per member (three to eight directors) or $350 per member (nine or more directors).

The Best Books

- *Boards That Make a Difference* by John Carver (San Francisco: Jossey-Bass, 1990). To order, call 800–956–7739.

  John Carver has produced a series of "CarverGuides" on a variety of governance topics. Sample titles: *Basic Principles of Policy Governance, Your Roles and Responsibilities as a Board Member, Three Steps to Fiduciary Responsibility, The Chairperson's Role as Servant-Leader* to the Board, Planning Better Board Meetings, Creating a Mission That Makes a Difference, Board Assessment of the CEO, Board Self-Assessment, and Making Diversity Meaningful in the Board Room. They cost $10.95 each and are available from Jossey-Bass; to order, call 800–956–7739.

- *The Future of Health Care Governance* by James E. Orlikoff and Mary K. Totten (Chicago: American Hospital Publishing, 1996).

  To order, call 800–242–2626.

- *Really Governing: How Health System and Hospital Boards Can Make More of a Difference* by Dennis D. Pointer and Charles M. Ewell (Albany, N.Y.: Delmar, 1994).

  To order, call 800–347–7707.

References and Bibliography

Alexander, J. A. "Governance for Whom? The Dilemmas of Change and Effectiveness in Hospital Boards." *Frontiers in Health Services Management,* Spring 1990, pp. 38–46.

Alexander, J. A. "Hospital Governance: Problems and Prospects for Health Services Research." *Journal of Health Administration Education,* 1992, 9, 395–424.

American Hospital Association Center for Healthcare Leadership and Ernst & Young, LLP. *1997 Hospital and Health System Governance Survey: Shining Light on Your Board's Passage to the Future.* Chicago: American Hospital Publishing, 1997.

Barker, J. A. *Paradigms: The Business of Discovering the Future.* New York: HarperBusiness, 1993.

"The Best and Worst Boards: Special Report on Corporate Governance." *Business Week,* Dec. 8, 1997.

Bowen, W. G. *Inside the Board Room.* New York: Wiley, 1993.

Carver, J. *Boards That Make a Difference: A New Design for Leadership in Nonprofit and Public Organizations.* San Francisco: Jossey-Bass, 1991.

Carver, J. *Boards That Make a Difference: A New Design for Leadership in Nonprofit and Public Organizations.* (2nd ed.) San Francisco: Jossey-Bass, 1997.

Carver, J., and Carver, M. M. *CarverGuide 1: Basic Principles of Policy Governance.* San Francisco: Jossey-Bass, 1996.

Carver, J., and Carver, M. M. *Reinventing Your Board: A Step-by-Step Guide to Implementing Policy Governance.* San Francisco: Jossey-Bass, 1997.

Chait, R. P., and Taylor, B. E. "Charting the Territory of Nonprofit Boards." *Harvard Business Review,* Jan. 1989, pp. 44–54.

Chait, R. P., and others. *The Effective Board of Trustees*. New York: Macmillan, 1991.

Chait, R. P., and others. *Improving Board Performance*. Phoenix, Ariz.: Oryx Press, 1993.

Coddington, D. C., and others. *Integrated Health Care: Reorganizing the Hospital, Physician and Health Plan Relationship*. Englewood, Colo.: Center for Research in Ambulatory Health Care Administration, Medical Group Management Association, 1994.

Collins, J. C., and Porras, J. "Building Your Company's Vision." *Harvard Business Review*, Sept.-Oct. 1996, pp. 65–77.

Deming, W. E. *Out of Crisis*. Cambridge, Mass.: MIT Press, 1982.

Doyle, M., and Straus, D. *How to Make Meetings Work: The New Interaction Method*. New York: Berkley Books, 1993.

Drucker, P. F. *Management: Tasks, Responsibilities, Practices*. New York: Harper-Collins, 1974.

Fox, W. M. *Effective Group Problem Solving: How to Broaden Participation, Improve Decision Making, and Increase Commitment to Action*. San Francisco: Jossey-Bass, 1987.

Frank, M. O. *How to Run a Successful Meeting in Half the Time*. New York: Pocket Books, 1989.

Geene, H. S. "Why Directors Can't Protect the Shareholders." *Fortune*, 1984, *110*, 28–29.

Hageman, W. M., and Umbdenstock, R. J. "Organizing and Focusing the Board's Work: Keys to Effectiveness." *Frontiers of Health Services Management*, 1990, 6, 29–46.

Holland, T., and others. *Improving Board Effectiveness: Practical Lessons for Non-profit Healthcare Organizations*. Chicago: American Hospital Publishing, 1997.

Houle, C. O. *Governing Boards: Their Nature and Nurture*. San Francisco: Jossey-Bass, 1989.

Kieffer, G. D. *The Strategy of Meetings*. New York: Warner Books, 1988.

Kotter, J. P. *Leading Change*. Boston: Harvard Business School Press, 1996.

Kouzes, J. M., and Posner, B. Z. *The Leadership Challenge: How to Keep Getting Extraordinary Things Done in Organizations*. San Francisco: Jossey-Bass, 1995.

Kuhn, T. S. *The Structure of Scientific Revolutions*. Chicago: University of Chicago Press, 1970.

Merry, M. D. *Professional Staff Credentialing*. La Jolla, Calif.: Governance Institute, 1994.

Molinari, C., and others. "The Effects of CEO-Board Relations on Hospital Performance." *Health Care Management Review*, 1997, *22* (3), 7–15.

Morrison, I. *The Second Curve: Managing the Velocity of Change.* New York: Ballantine, 1996.

Nanus, B. *Visionary Leadership: Creating a Compelling Sense of Direction for Your Organization.* San Francisco: Jossey-Bass, 1992.

Orlikoff, J. E. "Trouble in the Boardroom: The Seven Deadly Sins of Ineffective Governance." *Healthcare Forum Journal*, 1997, *40* (3), 38–42.

Orlikoff, J. E. *Quality from the Top: Working with Hospital Governing Boards to Assure Quality.* Chicago: Pluribus Press, 1990.

Orlikoff, J. E., and Totten, M. K. *The Board's Role in Quality Care: A Practical Guide for Hospital Trustees.* Chicago: American Hospital Publishing, 1991.

Orlikoff, J. E., and Totten, M. K. "Trustee Workbook: Board Composition and Trustee Selection." *Trustee*, Oct. 1995, unnumbered insert.

Orlikoff, J. E., and Totten, M. K. *The Future of Health Care Governance: Redesigning Boards for a New Era.* Chicago: American Hospital Publishing, 1996.

Orlikoff, J. E., and Totten, M. K. *The Trustee Handbook for Health Care Governance.* Chicago: American Hospital Publishing, 1998.

Pointer, D. D. "Really Governing: What Type of Work Should Boards Be Doing?" *Hospital and Health Services Administration*, 1995, *40* (3), 315–331.

Pointer, D. D. *Governance Trends and Practices: 1995 Panel Survey of Health System Boards.* La Jolla, Calif.: Governance Institute, 1995.

Pointer, D. D. *Governance Trends and Practices: 1996 Panel Survey of Hospital Boards.* La Jolla, Calif.: Governance Institute, 1996.

Pointer, D. D., and Ewell, C. M. *Really Governing: How Health System and Hospital Boards Can Make More of a Difference.* Albany, N.Y.: Delmar, 1994.

Pointer, D. D., Zuckerman, H., and Alexander, J. A. "Loosening the Gordian Knot of Governance in Integrated Health Care Delivery Systems." *Frontiers of Health Services Management*, Spring 1995, *11* (3), 3–38.

Pound, J. "The Promise of the Governed Corporation." *Harvard Business Review*, Mar.-Apr. 1993, pp. 89–98.

Senge, P. M. *The Fifth Discipline: The Art and Practice of the Learning Organization.* New York: Doubleday/Currency, 1990.

Shortell, S. M., Morrison, E. M., and Friedman, B. *Strategic Choices for America's Hospitals: Managing Change in Turbulent Times.* San Francisco: Jossey-Bass, 1990.

Shortell, S. M., and others. *Remaking Health Care in America: Building Organized Delivery Systems.* San Francisco: Jossey-Bass, 1996.

Smith, D. H. *Entrusted: The Moral Responsibilities of Trusteeship.* Bloomington: Indiana University Press, 1995.

Sofaer, S., and others. "What Do We Really Know About the Effect of Boards on Nonprofit Hospital Performance?" *Journal of Health Administration Education,* 1992, 9, 425–442.

Taylor, B. E., and others. "The New Work of the Nonprofit Board." *Harvard Business Review,* Sept.-Oct. 1996, pp. 4–11.

Wood, M. M. *Nonprofit Boards and Leadership: Cases on Governance, Change, and Board-Staff Dynamics.* San Francisco: Jossey-Bass, 1996.

Index